REACH
for
FITNESS

Other books by the author

RICHARD SIMMONS' BETTER BODY BOOK
RICHARD SIMMONS' NEVER-SAY-DIET BOOK
RICHARD SIMMONS' NEVER-SAY-DIET COOKBOOK

REACH
for
FITNESS

A special book of exercises for
the physically challenged

RICHARD SIMMONS

WARNER BOOKS

A Warner Communications Company

Richard Simmons Reach Foundation
is a California public benefit corporation

Exercise clothing provided by NIKE.
Wheelchairs provided by Everest & Jennings.
Text photographs by Bill Robbins.

Printed in the United States of America
First Printing: April 1986
10 9 8 7 6 5 4 3 2 1

Library of Congress Cataloging-in-Publication Data

Simmons, Richard.
    Reach for fitness.

    1. Physical fitness for the physically handicapped.
2. Exercise. 3. Nutrition. I. Title.
GV482.7.S56 1986   613.7′088081   85-43168
ISBN 0-446-51302-4

Designed by Giorgetta Bell McRee

*in memory of my loving father, who now
exercises with Bernie*

ACKNOWLEDGMENTS

I want you to know something about the people who spent over a year helping me bring this dream to life:

Nansey Neiman, Publisher, and Laurence J. Kirshbaum, President, Warner Books: It's very hard for a publisher to look at a great book idea and not see dollar signs. But when I approached Nansey and Larry about *Reach for Fitness,* they had such love and goodness in their hearts that they donated all profits to the Reach Foundation.

As Larry said, "It would be an honor for Warner Books to be associated with something this important."

Lawrence Apodaca, Executive Director, Reach Foundation: Several years ago I received a letter from a social worker at Orthopaedic Hospital in Los Angeles. Larry Apodaca told me that he had rewritten my book *Never Say Diet* so it would directly relate to his physically challenged clients. Later we talked about my dream for nutrition classes and exercise studios for the *handicapable.* It was Larry who nudged me until I got to work on the book you're holding in your hands.

Sam Britten, Ph.D., R.P.T., Director, Center of Achievement for the Physically Disabled, California State University at Northridge: I have never met a more sincere, dedicated, and hardworking human being. Besides that, Sam is a real pioneer in the science of nutrition and exercise for the physically challenged. He gave us years of experience and months of work when he helped us develop our exercise program.

Lynn Lee, R.P.T., Assistant Director of Therapies, Orthopaedic Hospital: Lynn is a wonderful, caring health professional who primarily works with handicapable children. During the photo sessions for this book, she patiently and gently taught the

Reach exercises to our models. More important, she made sure that all of the exercise instructions are clearly stated and *safe.*

Jack Turman, R.P.T., staff therapist at Orthopaedic Hospital: Jack is very knowledgeable in childhood diseases and he worked many long hours helping us develop our exercises.

Tim Green, Exercise Coordinator, Reach Foundation: Tim has so much energy and enthusiasm that people sometimes mistake him for my illegitimate son! He's a gymnast and an award-winning aerobics instructor whose love for people and pure joy of life are at the heart of our exercise program. Tim was also there during our photo sessions, keeping our energies up and making sure you saw how much fun we were having!

Bill Robbins, Photographer: What a remarkable man. You've all seen Bill's work on album covers and in magazines. He usually asks for and deserves top dollar for his art. But when I asked him to do the photos for this book for free, there was no hesitation. At one time in his life Bill was totally deaf (hearing has been restored in one ear), and he knew then that keeping his body in shape literally meant his survival. What he sees through his lens will now help you stay alive, too!!

Photographs for this book presented some real technical challenges for Bill's staff, and so I also want to thank Bill's studio manager, Alan Shaffer.

Linda Perigo Moore, Writer: Linda worked as my collaborator taking my thoughts and arranging them in the sentences and paragraphs you see here. The medical research on this project was staggering, and for more than a year Linda interviewed hundreds of doctors, therapists, and scientists about nutrition and exercise as they affect people with physical challenges. She worked so hard that I'm sure she could quit journalism, go before a medical board, and become an honorary doctor of something!

Nothing you see here could have materialized without the work of another very, very smart man. Thank you, to my manager, Stephen Miny. Stephen juggled a thousand details from other commitments so that I could spend valuable time on this project.

I'd also like to thank the following people for helping me understand some of the unique exercise and nutritional needs of people with physical challenges:

The Professional Advisory Committee of the Reach Foundation:

- R. Clark Davis, M.D.
- Alice Boylen, M.D.
- Rosalie Kane, D.S.W.
- Sam Britten, Ph.D.
- Richard Reese, Ph.D.
- Linda Lifur Bennett, Ph.D.

- Aubrey H. Fine, Ph.D.
- Mike Fawbush, M.A.
- Gordon Imlay, Ph.D.
- Stephen Snyder, M.D.
- Betty R. Wilson, Adm. Asst.

Catherine Baird of the California Governor's Committee for Employment of the Handicapped, Media Office, Sacramento, CA

Maureen E. Gaffney, R.N., M.N.
Freeman Memorial Hospital
Inglewood, CA

Leslie Shirakawa
Exceptional Children
    Foundation
Los Angeles, CA

Clive E. Brewster
Kerlan-Jobe Orthopedic
    Clinic
Inglewood, CA

Ann Fitzgerald
Access Project
Berkeley, CA

Ann Marie McGlynn
San Leandro, CA

Wilma Bower and
    Hildegarde Willard
Sacramento, CA

Laurie MacDonald, R.D.
Chief Clinical Dietitian
Orthopaedic Hospital
Los Angeles, CA

Wendy J. Parry
Children's Developmental
    Fitness Center
Pasadena, CA

Joan M. Saari
Vinland National Center
Loretto, MN

Sis Theuerkauf
Lakeshore Center
Birmingham, AL

Donald Comfort
Novato, CA

Cynthia Mercer
Los Angeles, CA

Marilynn Gay Montgomery
Pasadena, CA

OrthopædicHospital

Orthopaedic Hospital
2400 S. Flower Street
Los Angeles, CA 90007

Robert Sloane, President and Chief Executive Officer

This book and the work of the Reach Foundation are a reality because of the guidance, support, and dedication of the administrators and staff of Orthopaedic Hospital, Los Angeles.

My deepest and most sincere
Thank You,

Richard Simmons

FOREWORD

Since the dawn of time, man has always been faced with one challenge or another whether it be small or life threatening. He has always had to rise to the occasion to survive.

On this earth there are many people that have to face extraordinary challenges every day of their lives to merely exist in this hectic world.

This book is a wonderful testament to the inner strength and courage of handicapped adults and children that wish to excel in life. This guideline is a wonderful presentation on how much better one can make his life through discipline, dedication, and the pursuit of happiness.

Richard Simmons has opened the door that many thought impossible to open. Now it's just a matter of those brave enough to walk through and experience the exhilarating feeling of new self worth and pride.

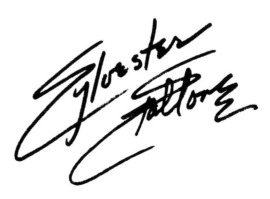

CONTENTS

REACH
for
FITNESS

PREFACE

I was a "handicapped" child. During my first eight years of school, I spent P.E. class sitting on a green bench watching everyone else toss the football, slide into base, and take home trophies for the top of the television set. I was not alone. Bernie was there, too. Bernie was in a wheelchair 'cause his legs didn't work and one of his arms was a little confused about what to do. We were both made fun of a lot—me because of my chubby body, steel-wool hair, and overdeveloped mouth, and Bernie because of his physical disabilities. We went through our own kind of hell because our "packaging" was different from the other kids'. (That's what faces and bodies are, you know, just packaging.)

I went through those school years never understanding why people like me and Bernie were ignored, put down, and made fun of. And from what I could tell, the grown-up world was no better. Adults in "different" packaging also experienced the same stares, looks, and unfair, even inferior, treatment.

This book is my way of telling Bernie that I've never forgotten him. *Reach for Fitness* is the very first book of exercise, nutrition, and fun for people who are physically (and/or medically) challenged.

If you're using a wheelchair or leg braces, if you have a progressive illness, or if you're in constant pain and discomfort, you may think that exercise classes and "building a body beautiful" are for "other people." Well, my friend, you're wrong. You need exercise and proper nutrition a thousand times more than those body-beautiful types. You need it for survival. Because your body has *special stresses,* those biological systems that are functioning must be *better* and *stronger.* Just plain "normal" isn't good enough. If you have a physical challenge, you have to know up front that exercise and nutrition are the best insurance policies you can have.

Exercise and proper nutrition can

strengthen and tone up your "working parts" so that you can more easily handle day-to-day living (all of those "simple little tasks" a lot of other people take for granted). They can also:

- assist in your physical rehabilitation,
- sometimes improve your medical treatments, and
- make you feel better 'cause it's so much fun.

BUT WHAT IF YOU'RE **NOT** PHYSICALLY CHALLENGED?

Maybe your own health is not the issue. Even so, you can still benefit from my plan of exercise and nutrition. You can read this book for someone else. For instance:

—IF as a new parent you've been told that your baby will have a disability and that not all of *your* experiences will come straight from the glossy photos in *New Baby Digest.*

—IF in the midst of career and child-rearing you've learned that your mother will never fully recover from that stroke she had last month.

—IF you extend yourself a little and share the message of this book with anybody you know who has a physical challenge.

Maybe you still don't recognize yourself. Maybe you're thinking, "I'm not handicapped and I don't know anybody who is." Maybe all you know about people with physical challenges is that they use handrails in public bathrooms and have parking spaces next to the front doors of stores. That doesn't matter, 'cause I've also written this book for *you.*

Ride in an automobile, fly down a ski slope, or walk up a wheelchair ramp and you can recognize the physical vulnerability of us all. You may be fine now— you have all of your limbs and they all work perfectly. That's wonderful, but nobody knows what's gonna happen next. Life is a gift; every day is like a Broadway show. When the curtain goes up and you step out there on that stage, you don't know if you're gonna be hit by a Sara Lee truck or what.

And so no matter why you've come here, you can also find encouragement and example. You can learn to reach out to someone else; you can learn how to help someone stretch his or her physical goals beyond anyone's expectations; and you can learn a lot about *strength* and *accomplishment.*

HOW DID THIS BOOK GET STARTED?

For the last decade I've been helping people like themselves better. I've been helping them look in their mirrors and see the strong, beautiful people inside the packaging. After I established my network of Anatomy Asylum exercise studios, I learned that it wasn't just the overweight people who had no place to go to exercise. There was another group of people who also had no place to develop themselves to their full physical potential. And so as my life's work has evolved, I haven't just focused on the people with a few extra fat cells; I've also focused on the people, like Bernie, who may have a progressive illness or who may have a limb that just didn't turn out "perfect."

No one was ever turned away from any of my exercise classes. When a hospital asked me to come and exercise senior citizens or children with Down's syndrome or just "motivate my guts out" for anybody—I went.

After five years of screaming down the corridors of hundreds of hospitals, I was asked to become the national spokesperson for spina bifida. (Don't feel bad if you don't know what that is—at first I thought it was a children's cereal!)

My work with the Spina Bifida Association led to requests to serve on boards and special commissions for numerous health organizations. Suddenly, I had a chance to learn three new and very important lessons:

1. There are VERY FEW well-equipped, fun-filled exercise facilities for people with disabilities.
2. Such facilities cost a lot a money.
3. You can get money for these projects by begging for it or by raising it.

I decided to raise it!

I went to my editors at Warner Books and told them that I wanted to write a book for people who thought they had good excuses for not exercising. Then I told them that I wanted to put my royalties into a foundation that would build exercise facilities for these same people. They said, "Richard, you set up that foundation and you can have our profits, too."

And so the Reach Foundation was born. This not-for-profit organization has the primary purpose of creating community- and hospital-based exercise studios for people with disabilities. We're not interested in reproducing clinics or therapy rooms. Our studios will be full of mirrors, music, bright-colored lights, and the excitement of personal accomplishment. (I mean, just because you have a problem moving doesn't mean that you have to be GRIM!)

Every Reach studio will be staffed by people with physical challenges. And so in addition to creating a revolutionary exercise environment, we are also employing the skills of some pretty remarkable people who, frankly, have had trouble getting jobs in the "open market."

As we grow, we also have plans for nutrition and health education classes for parents and children. And our ultimate goal is to offer job skills training and placement for people with disabilities.

This project has already taken several years and millions of words. First, I gathered together a team of people dedicated to my dream and they became the foundation's advisory committee. Next, we selected an administrative officer and mailed out hundreds of questionnaires to health care professionals and individuals with physical challenges. Representatives from all major areas of medicine and rehabilitation, as well as the heads of charitable organizations representing specific illnesses and disabilities, were contacted. Eighty-three doctors; over 100 physical therapists, social workers, psychologists, nutritionists, and nurses; and dozens of "handicapable" individuals have contributed (as in "have volunteered and given") to this project.

As you hold this book in your hands, you are holding their time, sweat, love, and work. And the theoretical basis of our program did not come about through research with laboratory mice. Rather, our concepts and our methods come from real human beings who meet physical challenges every day of their lives. (You'll see some of them later as we demonstrate our exercises.)

ALL profit from every book sold anywhere will be put into the Reach Foundation and used to extend physical confidence to lots of folks who may have given up on their bodies. (Can you see what's happened here? You've already helped the Reach Foundation by simply buying this book! Now, how about buying a few more—as gifts for your friends and relatives? We can make a deal on bulk mailings!!)

Reach for Fitness has two main goals:

My first goal is for the person with a physical and/or medical challenge. I want you to learn how you can join those handicapable individuals who practice regular exercise and good nutrition *in spite of* what everyone else calls a handicap. I want you to learn more about your body—what to feed it and how to move it. And I want you to love the improvements you're gonna see.

My second goal is for all of you who are called able-bodied. I want you to re-evaluate the ways you probably judge "the handicapped." I want you to look beyond the wheelchair ramps and the yearly telethons. Most of all, I want you to start looking at everybody with love and respect—not pity. People with physical challenges are just like everyone else. They don't want your pity—they want acceptance. And they want the excitement of personal accomplishment!

The best way to achieve this is with knowledge. But until a physical challenge touches our own lives, few of us know anything about it. We don't know the names of illnesses, or which ones have cures. We don't realize that most people who have physical disabilities are in no way medically ill. We don't think about things like how people in wheelchairs have to shift around constantly or they get sore bottoms. Or that a kid who will not live to adulthood still has a right to a childhood. Most of the time we don't know what to say or what not to say or where to rest our eyes when we talk to someone who cannot control the muscles in his face. In this, the most educated country on Earth, the whole subject is still in the shadows. And so the first thing we want to do for you is to shed a little light. In our appendix, you will find out how medical experts define over forty illnesses and physical disabilities and what they say about the effects of exercise upon rehabilitation. Just read one appendix entry a night and you'll be a changed person.

I went to a Catholic school (Our Lady of Perpetual Repentance), and the nuns were always repeating that old adage: "I cried because I had no shoes until I saw a man who had no feet." I think this was supposed to make us feel humble and grateful for our blessings. But it always upset me. I couldn't stop wondering about that man with no feet. Did the adage mean that the footless man was hopeless? No, it couldn't be! Did it mean that if something happened to my feet (personally, I have lousy feet) then I, too, would be hopeless?? Again, a thousand times NO! He may have had no feet, I'd always conclude, but he could've had a brilliant mind and an open heart. Once I recognized that this man in my teachers' example was capable of fantastic accomplishment, then I wasn't afraid anymore. And that's why most of us so-called able-bodied are ignorant about the disabled world. We think that if we ignore it, it'll never include us! We at the Reach Foundation know that those fears are wasted energy—'cause *anybody* can make what he has better, no matter what.

So now you know our story, our goals, and how we've developed this program of exercise, nutrition, and information. All I can say to you at this point is thank you. Thank you for picking up this book, and thank you for putting down your hard cash. You know where that money's going, and after you read this book, I know that *you'll* be going in the right direction. If you've let your body get fat and weak because you thought of yourself as hopeless or if you've ignored the challenges and accomplishments of others—it's time to grow.

CHAPTER 1

For All You Do— This Book's for You

The whole world's exercising! Everywhere you look, legs are jogging, buns are bouncing, hands are reaching, stretching, pulling.... And you can't do it, right? You use a wheelchair. Or your arthritis acts up every other Tuesday. Or you've lost a limb. Or you have multiple sclerosis. Or you just don't feel up to it. Anyway, you look terrible in your orthopedic leotard—and, besides, nobody expects you to shape up, 'cause you just can't....

HOLD IT!! Do not read *another* word until you repeat after me:

I, _____, have picked up this book because deep in my heart I know that every living, breathing cell in my body (even those that don't work so good right now)—that every living cell in my body could be better, stronger, and healthier with a little concentrated activity. Therefore, I solemnly swear that I will NEVER, EVER again say that I CAN'T exercise! So help me, God. Amen.

This book is the first of its kind. Never before has there been such a universal exercise and nutrition plan for children and adults with polio, spina bifida, asthma, cerebral palsy, cystic fibrosis, spinal cord injury, muscular dystrophy, kidney disease, multiple sclerosis, or any other condition that limits mobility. And yet, people who don't move tend to get FAT. Obesity (a polite word for fat) ranks as the number one complication for all of these medical and physical challenges. Even if you escape FAT, a lack of physical activity will cause those unaffected muscles to atrophy, or waste away. This could be your chance to beat the odds. But maybe you still need convincing. Take the following self-analysis and see if you recognize anybody. Then we'll talk turkey (hold the mayo).

THE DO-I-REALLY-NEED-THIS-GRIEF QUIZ

(Check each truthful statement. No fibbing!)

— The only veggies I ever eat are the pickles on my cheeseburger.

— When we go shopping, my friends have stopped asking me to tote their packages. The wheelchair's already full.

— I spend a lot of time anticipating my next meal.

— When I go to the grocery, my braces ice up from leaning against the Sealtest freezer.

— I've graduated from a size Husky to a Pre-Cabana.

— Sure, I use crutches. But that's never stopped me from spending the seventh-inning stretch balancing a Coney dog, a beer, popcorn, cotton candy, and a chocolate Slurpee.

— My idea of exercise is going through the brunch buffet instead of ordering from the menu.

— When I go to a salad bar, I usually eat the chocolate pudding and the canned peaches.

— I'm POSITIVE that Twinkies can cure headaches.

— Exercise makes me wheeze, but I can still walk to the fridge for a frozen Snickers.

Scoring:

1-2 items checked—Give this book to a friend who needs it.

3-6 items checked—Don't worry. We're having this little meeting just in time.

7-10 items checked—If I were you, I'd make notes in the margins.

You've seen your score—it's time to stop making excuses. Start planning an exercise program this very minute or you'll find yourself being carted off to an early grave. A grave that you've dug with your own dessert spoon.

By now you're probably wondering just how **I've got the nerve** to tell you that you have no excuse for not exercising!! What could *I* possibly know about *your* problems? And frankly, my dear,

why would I even give a damn? Well, give me a minute and I'll tell you why.

The world thinks that having a physical challenge means a world of wheelchairs, braces, and crutches. But there are a lot of things that can keep you from totally experiencing and enjoying life. I've never had to use a wheelchair, but I've been encased in a world of flesh that was just as restrictive. I have all of my limbs, but I know what it is when there's no easy way to move them or there's no place to hide them. And I know what it means to be stared at in pity. I know all of this because I have been FAT. But what I really know is how to *stop* being fat.

THIS IS IT! PUT YOUR TOKEN ON THE GAME BOARD

We're going to start by clearing away all of the labels. When we began this book, there was sincere concern among the participants in our project: "For God's sake, don't put the word 'handicapped' on the cover." "Use the word 'disabled,'" others insisted. "Words don't matter; every body deteriorates. We're all temporarily able-bodied (TABs), anyway." "It can't be done. You're bound to offend someone!"

What we have to accomplish is far too valuable to be lost in semantics. So we're going to move beyond that. Read the following list and pick a phrase that meets with your approval:

- Disabled
- Able-Disabled
- Handicapped
- Courageous
- Slightly Limited
- Physically Impaired
- Physically Challenged
- Disadvantaged
- Hanging in There
- Your own phrase

I don't want to offend you by calling you something that you don't like. So everytime I use a phrase that grates on

your nerves or distracts from my message, mark it out in your copy of the book. Just scratch right through it with a pencil or a bulldozer and write *your* phrase above it.

Now then, on to the more important matters—like our feelings about our bodies. First, I think that every one of us is at the same time both handicapped and handicapable. All those beautiful, successful, and vivacious people (you know, the ones who make you gag, they look so perfect!)—all of those people still have major flaws and weaknesses. (And I'm not talking pimples on their backs—I'm talking major stuff!) No human being escapes these things. Each of us struggles with *something*. And frankly, just because your problems may be more outwardly obvious doesn't automatically mean that you're worse off than anyone else. We're not into judgments here! I can't judge your pain or give it a score. Do you expect me to say: "On the big H.S. (Handicapped Scale), you get six points for wheelchair. You lose two points because you can still hobble around"? NO—that's silly! You're the only one who can give definition to those goals that *you* wish to accomplish as a result of reading this book. You're the only one who really knows what mountains you can and cannot move.

But at the same time, we are all *handicapable*. This is to say that we each have the inner strength necessary for remarkable accomplishment. So if you're a "seven," you can become a "seven and a half," and if you're a "three," you can become a "four." I believe this with all my heart and I see this truth every day of my life. The most obvious confirmation has come through my work on the Richard Simmons' TV program and in my Anatomy Asylum exercise studios.

Here I see thousands of transformations. They waddle in, miserable and self-conscious "threes or fours." After lots of hard work and even more sweat, they glide away as beautiful "tens."

Because of this success at motivating others to exercise and eat wisely, I've been invited into clinics and hospitals throughout the nation. People gather in wheelchairs, on crutches, and in braces. We turn on the music and we move. We move whatever it is that we *can* move— a neck or a toe. And the next time, we move a little more.

One particularly memorable session took place at Dr. Sam Britten's Center of Achievement for the Physically Disabled, California State University, Northridge. As I entered the room, people came over, joked, and generally made me feel at home. I turned to a young woman using a wheelchair, extended my hand, and said, "Hi. I'm Richard Simmons."

She looked at me with such disdain that every muscle in her face said, "So?" Then she whipped that chair a clean 180 degrees and wheeled to the opposite side of the room.

Sam put his hand on my back and said softly, "It's not you. Her accident was less than a year ago and she's still working through some of the initial anger. It'll be okay."

I began the session with this plea:

"The next time you reach for that candy bar or cake, please recite this pledge: 'I am a survivor. I am in control! And after all the grief and pain I've been through, I will not destroy my own body with this crap!!'"

We had a *fantastic* work-out—Laughing, stretching, dancing to the music. But "you know who" didn't join us. She just glared at me. What was she thinking? Was it just my presence that offended her? My face? My hair? Something I said? I'm not known for holding back, but, usually, people see that my honesty is only sincere concern for them—and so it's okay. It wasn't working with her. I had bombed. When one person in an audience rejects me, I find myself focusing in, trying even harder to reach out only to those eyes. Nothing.

The session ended. I hugged most everyone goodbye and headed home to soak my aching arches. As I was getting into my car, I saw her coming out of the building. She took a bag of chips from her book satchel. But instead of opening it, she slapped the bag to her lap, wheeled to a trash can, and dumped the whole mess. I could've floated home!

The love, determination, and just plain guts I've witnessed in sessions such as the one at Northridge have convinced me that exercise and nutrition can help *anyone.*

OUR GAME PLAN

Reach for Fitness is divided into three major sections: an EXERCISE and FOOD 4 LIFE program for adults, an EXERCISE and FOOD 4 LIFE program for children, and the medical appendix. This way you can focus on those motivational, dietary, and physical factors most appropriate to your needs.

In each of the first two sections, you will find:

exercises for specific body areas: head to tush to toe,
a volume food plan, and
hints on how to develop a system of mental control.

Finally, but most important, the book contains an appendix of medical conditions and physical challenges. Unlike reading other books, you should go to this section first!! We're not talking about literary leftovers or bibliographies that nobody ever looks up anyway. Here you will find advice from experts in physical therapy, medicine, nursing, occupational therapy, psychology, and nutrition regarding the *specific* dos and don'ts of your individual EXERCISE and FOOD 4 LIFE program.

YOUR GAME PLAN

Step 1: Read the appendix.

Step 2: Identify parts of your body that need attention now.

Step 3: Show the book and your choices to your doctor. (I really spruced up for these pictures, so you can take me anywhere!)

Step 4: LIVE.

CHAPTER 2

Why It's Gonna Work This Time

(A short chapter, but very meaningful.)

Put down this book and go over to your bookcase....

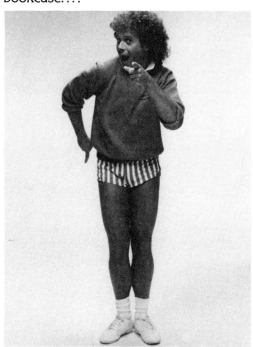

I knew you'd be back, 'cause you didn't wait for me to finish my sentence.

When you get to the bookcase, pull out a diet book. I'm sure you've got one 'cause I read somewhere that there're approximately 27.4 diet books for every man, woman, and child in America. There're more diet books than toothbrushes and almost more diet books than croissants in these very United States!

Got it? It doesn't matter which one (the low-protein, high-protein, low-carbohydrate, no-carbohydrate, the fiber-fill, or the fast), they all say the same thing:

"You may not eat _____ for _____ weeks, and then you get to be like a real person again."

You can *lose* weight on any of these plans (especially the one that has you eat crushed eggshells and herb tea for three days). But once lost, that weight usually follows a trail of breadcrumbs or something and finds its way back home to your thighs. This happens because of the basic psychology of the *special food, short-term* diet plan. What do you feel most like doing when you're on such a

D-I-E-T? D-I-E, right? As in: "I could just *die* for a piece of cheesecake!" Such short-term restrictions don't work because they don't teach you how to LIVE with food. So as soon as you go back to "normal" eating, you quickly regain lost weight.

The only rival for a diet book is a celebrity exercise book. If King Kong could tell us how he had the strength to carry Fay Wray up the Empire State Building, then, believe me, he'd have an exercise book, too.

But exercise programs can be just as temporary. Maybe you've tried, I mean, *really* tried exercise. You've tried and yet you're still flabby. You got an exercise book, you worked long enough to get sore, and then it was over. Or maybe you bought one of those weight-loss gadgets you see on TV. (Trust me, Saran Wrap girdles will not firm up your waistline.) Now, you may look at these past experiences and consider yourself a failure. All the promises you've made about what you were going to do with your body—none of these have materialized. Well, it's time to stop feeling sorry for yourself.

Whether you're in a wheelchair or out of a wheelchair, you don't FAIL at diets or exercise programs, you just QUIT. If you had ever continued on with any diet or exercise routine, then you wouldn't have this problem right now.

What I want you to do today is to erase all of the negative feelings you have about past exercise and food programs and start fresh.

Just like anybody else, it's gonna take you three steps to get into shape:

1. You're going to have to learn how to exercise your body.
2. You're going to have to learn how to eat. (And usually, that means *less*.)
3. You're going to have to learn how to be a self-motivator.

Maybe you failed in previous exercise or food plans because you never learned to keep your goal in mind and to motivate yourself on a DAILY basis. But in the following chapters, we're gonna teach you how to finally get it all together.

CHAPTER 3

EXERCISE 4 LIFE:
A Program for Adults

This is it! You're ready to start moving that body of yours in ways that are going to *amaze* you.

A couple of pointers before we begin:

The most important thing now is that you set realistic goals. Don't enter your exercise program thinking that it's one of those Mr. or Ms. Muscle contests. A better goal is to achieve and maintain overall body fitness with exercises that require you to stretch, relax, flex, and move your muscles and joints as much as you can.

As you approach each exercise, remember that nobody's keeping score. This is not a sport—there is no competition—you're not gonna get a washer and dryer or a trip to Paris if you win. If everyone else is doing ten repetitions of an exercise and you can only do five, then do five good ones. After all, isn't doing five better than doing *none?* Stop comparing your body to anybody else's.

Just trust me, you'll know when you're ready for more. And after you start feeling better about what your body can do, you'll want more!

THE SUCCESSFUL EXERCISER'S CREDO

If you exercise once a week, it's about as helpful as falling out of a window. If you exercise twice a week, you'll be maintaining your body at its present level. But research shows that if you exercise at least every other day you will see major change!

DEFINITION OF EXERCISE CATEGORIES

My friends and I will demonstrate four different exercise categories for every area of your body. Some will be less difficult for you to practice; some will be more difficult or even inappropriate. This is why you must carefully analyze your physical needs and challenges and then select only those exercises that will be of most benefit for your *individual* body.

You will see that many of our exercises can begin in either a standing, sitting, or lying-down position. Pick the best starting position for you and evaluate that decision often. For example, you may begin an exercise in the sitting position and learn that with practice you can complete the same exercise while standing. During periods of medical or physical stress (temporary or progressive) you may even decide to do all of your exercises sitting or lying down. Where you do your exercises doesn't matter nearly as much as the fact that you *do* them.

The four exercise categories are: warm-up, isometric, isotonic and stretching/cool-down.

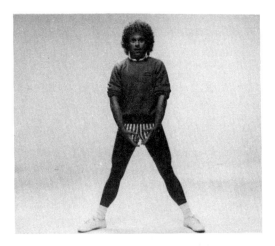
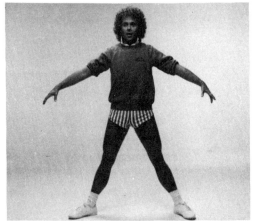
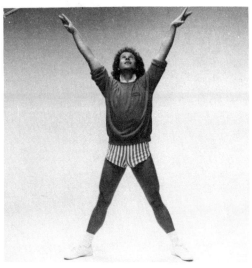

1. WARM-UP

In a warm-up exercise, you will move a joint through its full or partial range of motion. We use the term "range of motion" (ROM) a lot in this chapter, and it means something a little different for everybody. For example, for most of us, the ROM for a shoulder is a complete circle. But if you have something that restricts joint movement (something like arthritis), your shoulder's ROM may be only a small part of that circle. When an exercise instruction tells you to move a joint or muscle through its range of motion, that means you are to move as much as you can without pain. Your individual ROM may really improve with exercise, or it may be permanently impaired. In either case, you need to move every joint through its individual ROM *every single day!*

I'm sure you've heard the word "aerobic." It literally means "containing oxygen" and it refers to action in which your lungs, heart, and muscles use oxygen in the most efficient way possible. Steadily performing a warm-up exercise (usually for five to eight minutes) will create an aerobic exercise.

2. ISOMETRIC

Isometric is another exercise term you've probably used before, and it means pushing against something that doesn't move. Pushing against the door of the fridge so it won't open up and make you eat something is a good example of an isometric exercise.

Isometric exercises are especially terrific when you cannot move around or complete the more active warm-up exercises. This may not *look* like exercise, but when you do this pushing and resisting, you'll still *feel* your muscles working.

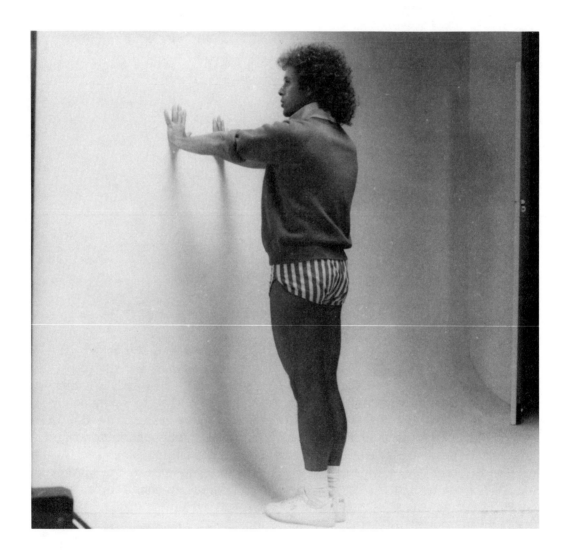

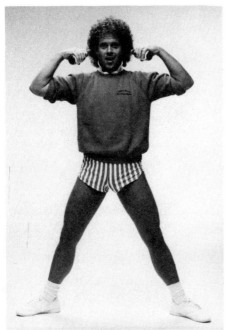

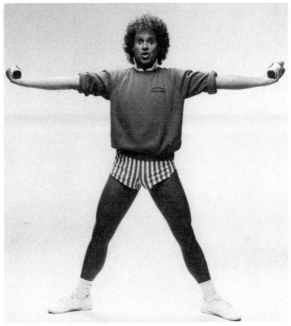

3. ISOTONIC

Isotonic may be a new word for you, but it simply means moving with a weighted object. So while you are moving those weights, you are also *moving* those muscles and related joints through their range of motion.

You can build bigger and stronger muscles if you increase the weight. (But start with small objects and *do not* increase the weight until you can cor-rectly complete at least twelve consecu-tive repetitions!)

Your weights don't have to be fancy gym equipment—household objects like books, canned goods, or pots and pans will do just as well. For example, you can start with something small, like a single-serving can of vegetables, and gradually move up to a family size econo-pac. Even if you have difficulty grasping a weighted object, you can get a similar benefit if someone else gently pushes against your movement.

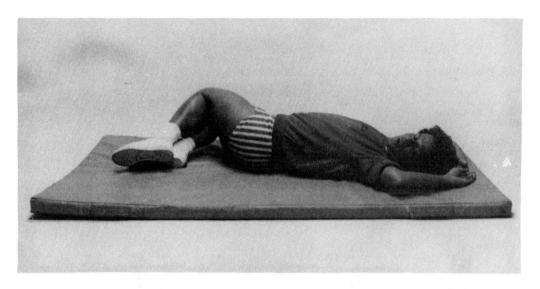

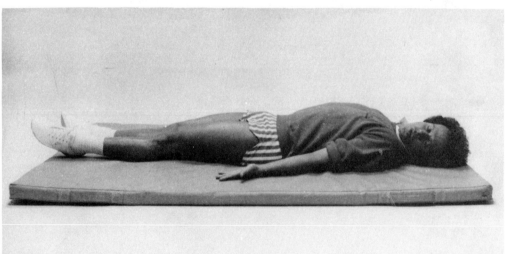

4. STRETCHING/ COOL-DOWN

After all of that warm-up, isometric, and isotonic action, you need to relax. And so the fourth type of exercise allows you to move joints and stretch muscles slowly

through their full or partial range. These relaxation and cool-down movements will help you increase joint mobility, decrease muscle soreness, and control involuntary muscle contractions (spasticity).

Besides, this is your reward for a "major work-out," and it feels *soooooo* good.

How The Exercises Are Organized

As you look through the exercise section, you'll see a very definite pattern. (We didn't just throw this stuff together, ya know.) Major muscle groups within your body have been assigned exercises from each of the four exercise categories, and we call this a "set." For example, an exercise set that works your shoulder muscles could consist of:

1. Shoulder Shrugs (SH5)—a warm-up exercise
2. Shoulder Presses (SH7)—an isometric exercise
3. Weighted Shoulder Shrugs (SH10)—an isotonic exercise
4. Shoulder Stretches (SH11)—a stretching/cool-down exercise.

Plan your exercise program in sets so that you never do an isometric exercise before warming up and never move on to a new muscle group before doing a stretching (or cool-down) exercise.

In previous books I've organized exercises into beginning, intermediate, and advanced programs. But that isn't possible here. Because each of you has unique physical challenges, you, your doctor, and your physical therapist must construct an *individualized* plan from the exercises we've designed. For example, if you have no control or movement in your hips and legs, you may construct an exercise program using the exercises for the neck, arms, and upper torso. If you have a disease that is now at a stressful stage, you can still get a fantastic work-out by doing the isometric exercises for each body part. And if you complete an hour of the warm-up exercises, you'll have yourself a dandy little aerobics program.

This brings me to the matter of repetitions. Most exercise books list a specific number of times you should repeat an exercise, but the amount of exercise you need is also something too individualized for us to predetermine. And so at the end of an exercise that should be repeated, you will see the phrase "repeat as able."

If you're not moving a muscle at all right now, then one contraction is a 100 percent improvement. But, if you don't have a physical restriction to movement and you've just been lazy, then start out with three to five repetitions and gradually add more as you improve. Everybody has limits. Know yours, but DON'T BABY YOURSELF. If you know that you are able to do something, don't make a lot of excuses. And always keep your goal in mind.

Finally, don't skip the relaxation/cool-down exercises. These are your reward for good work, but they also stretch and maintain muscles that have become tight because of inactivity.

Take a deep breath and . . .

You should begin each session with a little exercise in proper breathing. Oh, sure, you think you know how to breathe already, right? I mean, you've been doing it pretty good for a while now—what else do you need to learn?

EFFICIENT breathing—not just the kind that keeps you from falling over dead—begins when you take a slow, deep breath of air. The oxygen in that breath moves from your lungs, through your heart, and up and all over your brain cells. All of that fresh oxygen means that you feel better and you think better. (Just ask any of those Indian yogis—they're excellent breathers and they all say they think and feel fantastic!!) The second phase of efficient breathing occurs when you get rid of carbon dioxide, the waste product from all of that heart and lung action. (Remember your eighth-grade biology class? Animals use the oxygen, and plants use the carbon dioxide, 'cause God was very clever that way.)

Ready? Straighten your back as much as you can (sitting or standing, it doesn't matter). Eyes forward. (You have already blown your nose, right?) Begin.

Attention: Breathing Lesson in Progress

Most people let the muscles of their upper chest and neck control all of their breathing. This shallow kind of upper chest breathing is very inefficient and actually requires you to take in more oxygen than necessary. The muscle that should be controlling your breathing is the diaphragm, and it is located in that space below your ribs and above your navel. If you've been using shallow upper chest breathing, your diaphragm has grown weak and flabby. Time to shape it up.

Step One: Close your mouth and inhale through your nose. (If you open both your mouth and your nose as you inhale, you'll just sort of gag a little and sound like an *oink-oink.*)

As you bring in the air, concentrate upon filling your lungs as much as possible. You'll notice that as you inhale your diaphragm will push out your stomach to make room for your expanding lungs.

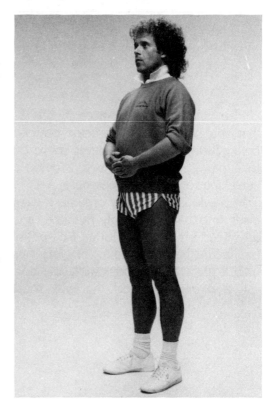

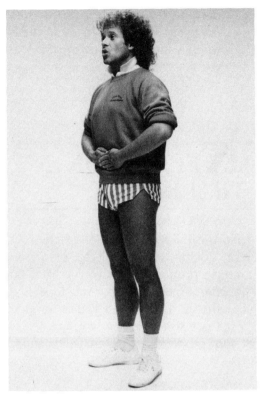

Step Two: Hold in all that air for a second or two. (Now quickly read Step Three.)

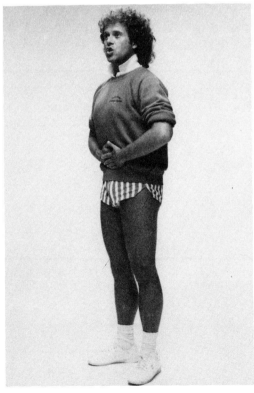

Step Three: Open your lips a little and let all of that air slowly and evenly glide out of your mouth. NOT SO FAST. As you exhale, pull in your stomach and help that diaphragm push the air out of your lungs.

Step Four: You think all the air's pushed out? Push your stomach in a little tighter. (You can even help it along by gently pressing your hands against your belly button.) Blow out that last molecule of carbon dioxide. Out . . . out . . . there's one more in there!

Step Five: Slowly inhale once more. (This last part is very important. Your friends would absolutely panic if they had to call the paramedics now.)

Finally, exercise and breathing should follow a rhythmic pattern:

1. As you flex a muscle (or at the beginning of a motion), close your mouth and breathe in through your nose. When you breathe in, you're gonna fill your stomach with so much air that it's gonna feel like you've just eaten Thanksgiving dinner at your grandmother's house.

2. As you relax a muscle (or at the end of a motion), breathe out through your mouth and use your diaphragm to PUSH out all of that hot air. (And God knows we're all full of hot air.)

3. Never hold your breath during any motion. In fact, if you don't breathe during your exercises, you will die. And it's real hard to look pretty when your face is turning blue as you're trying to do "one more leg lift."

KEEPING ON TRACK

Take the following "challenge chart" to your doctor and use it to plan your exercise program. After you've filled out the chart, make a copy and tape it to your fridge. Then when you're tempted to sneak a snack, look at your goal, look at your progress, and exercise instead!!

MY CHALLENGE CHART

Month: _____   Weight Goal: _____

Date: _____   Present Weight: _____   Date: _____   Present Weight: _____

    _____   _____   _____   _____

    _____   _____   _____   _____

    _____   _____   _____   _____

    _____   _____   _____   _____

	Exercise Name Page Number	Repetitions	Week One	Week Two	Week Three	Week Four	Week Five
WARM-UP Neck							
Shoulders							
Arms							
Hands							
Back							
Chest							
Waist & Stomach							
Hips & Buttocks							
Thighs							
Lower Legs							
Feet							
ISOMETRIC Neck	(no repetitions needed)						
Shoulders							
Arms							
Hands							
Back							
Chest							
Waist & Stomach							
Hips & Buttocks							
Thighs							
Lower Legs							
Feet							

	Exercise Name Page Number	Repetitions	Week One	Week Two	Week Three	Week Four	Week Five
ISOTONIC Neck							
Shoulders							
Arms							
Hands							
Back							
Chest							
Waist & Stomach							
Hips & Buttocks							
Thighs							
Lower Legs							
Feet							
STRETCHING/ COOL-DOWN Neck							
Shoulders							
Arms							
Hands							
Back							
Chest							
Waist & Stomach							
Hips & Buttocks							
Thighs							
Lower Legs							
Feet							

ONE REAL, HONEST-TO-GOODNESS WARNING

If it hurts—STOP. I'm not talking about the stiffness or mild aching you can expect the first couple of days of your new exercise program. That's normal. But if you experience serious discomfort or worsening of your medical symptoms, then check with your physician. You may simply need to reevaluate your plan and begin again with another type of exercise.

YOUR LAST CHECKPOINTS

(I promise, these are the very last ones and then we'll get to the good stuff!)

—— Check the appendix for any specific information about your particular physical and/or medical challenge.

—— Check out your exercise plan with your doctor.

—— Check for ice-cream bars still hiding in the freezer. (Don't forget to look behind those tubs of turkey broth you've been saving since Thanksgiving 1981.)

—— Check out your exercise environment so it's just the way you like it. Maybe a little music. Maybe some fresh air. Better yet, a friend.

—— Don't get discouraged. It's gonna be slow at first. That extra weight took time to pile up, so it's gonna take some time to get it off. Just remember that the work you put in now will come back to you a thousandfold.

YOU CAN DO IT. I KNOW YOU CAN!

Before we start, I'd like to mention some very important people who worked to develop the EXERCISE 4 LIFE program. They are:

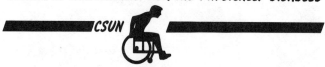

CENTER OF ACHIEVEMENT FOR THE PHYSICALLY DISABLED

CAL STATE UNIVERSITY NORTHRIDGE
Physical Education Department

18111 Nordhoff St.
Northridge, California 91330

Consultant:

Sam Britten, Ph.D.
—Director
    Center of Achievement for the Physically Disabled
    California State University, Northridge
    Northridge, CA

Consultant:

Peggy Lasko
—Director
    Fitness Center
        for the Physically Disabled
    San Diego, CA

Consultant:

Cathy Smith, M.A.
—Physical Therapist
    Los Angeles Unified School District
    Los Angeles, CA

OrthopædicHospital

**RICHARD SIMMONS'
REACH
FOUNDATION**

Orthopaedic Hospital • 2400 South Flower Street • Los Angeles, CA 90007 • (213) 742-1332

Consultants:

Lynn Lee, R.P.T.
—Assistant Director of
    Therapies

Jack Turman, R.P.T.,
—Staff Therapist
    Orthopaedic Hospital
    Los Angeles, CA

Tim Green
—Exercise Coordinator
    Reach Foundation
    Los Angeles, CA

THE MODELS APPEARING IN THIS CHAPTER ARE:

Darryn Bernard Brooks, actor.
Bernard is a person with traumatic incomplete paraplegia.

Ivy! Gunter, fashion model.
Ivy! is a person with a leg amputation as a result of cancer.

Gerry Jewel, actress and comedienne.
Gerry is a person with cerebral palsy.

Chris Templeton, actress.
Chris is a person with postpolio.

Alan Toy, actor.
Alan is a person with postpolio.

NECK

N1   Head Tilts

Position: standing or sitting, back straight, and eyes forward.
Type: Warm-up

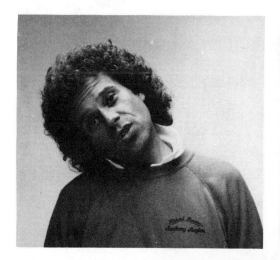 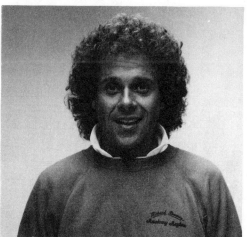

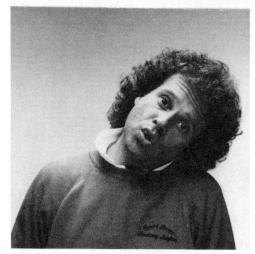

1. Slowly bend head toward right shoulder.
2. Return to starting position.
3. Now slowly bend head toward left shoulder.
4. Return to starting position and repeat as able.

Note: Practice in front of mirror the first time to be sure you don't twist your neck or turn your chin toward your shoulder.

N2   Side Head Presses

Position: standing or sitting.
Type: Isometric

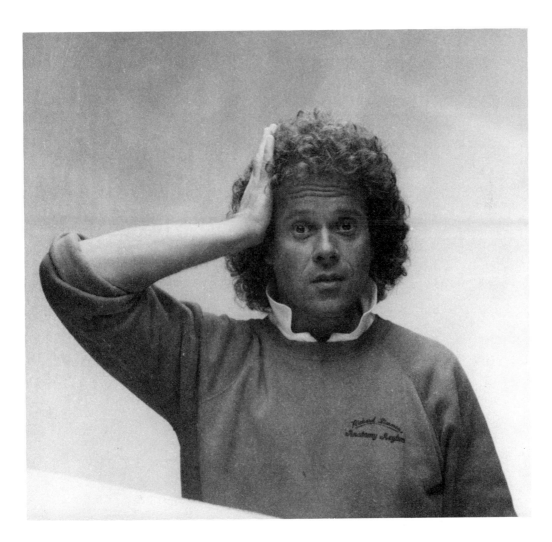

1. Place right hand against right side of head.
2. Using right hand to resist movement, try to bend head toward right shoulder. Hold for five seconds. Repeat as able.
3. Alternate sides and repeat as able.

Note: We don't want movement here—so you should be as still as I am in the picture!

N3 Moving Side Head Presses

Position: standing or sitting.
Type: Isotonic

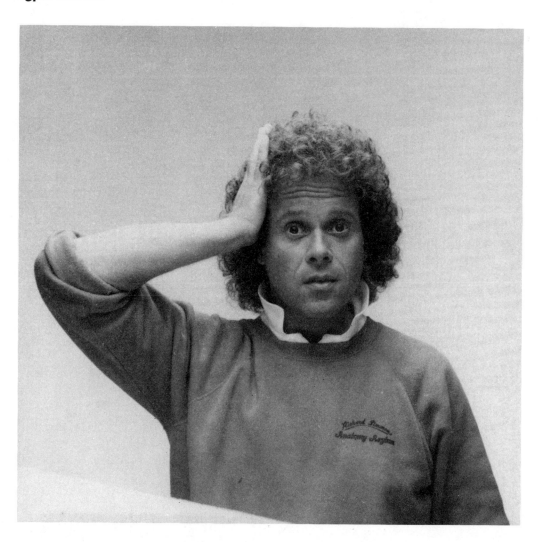

1. Place right hand against right temple.
2. Using hand to resist movement, slowly bend head toward right shoulder. Return to starting position and repeat as able.
3. Alternate sides and repeat as able.

Note: If you do not have independent control, do not allow anyone else to move your head through this exercise.

N4   See-Saws

Position: standing or sitting.
Type: Warm-up

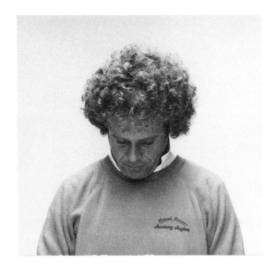
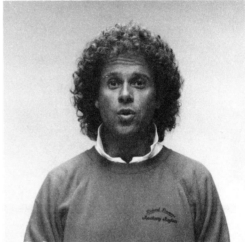

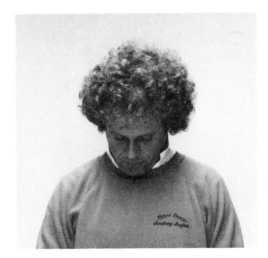

1. Slowly drop chin to chest. (Careful—it's not necessary to *smash* it down.)
2. Lift head up and look straight ahead.
3. Return to starting position and repeat as able.

N5 Front-Back Head Presses

Position: standing or sitting.
Type: Isometric

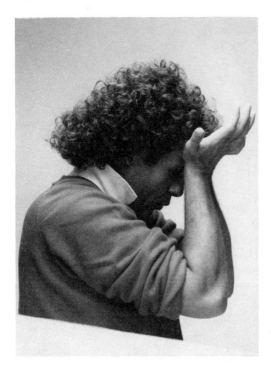

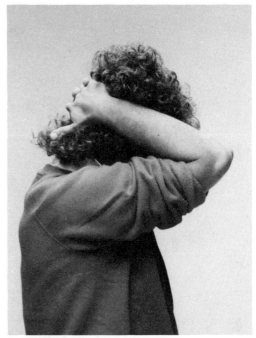

1. Place heel of both palms against your forehead and hold firmly.
2. Using palms to resist movement, press head forward and slightly downward. Hold for five seconds.
3. Return to starting position and lock hands on back of head (not neck). Hold firmly.
4. Using hands to resist movement, press head slightly upward. Hold for five seconds.

Note: Remember, no real motion should take place.

N6   Neck No-Nos

Position: standing or sitting, head erect, eyes forward.
Type: Warm-up

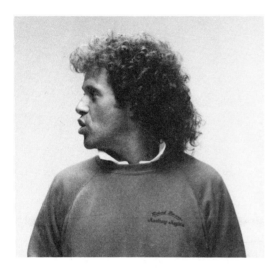 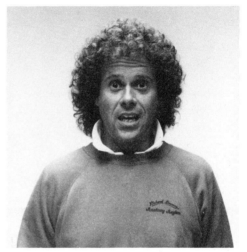

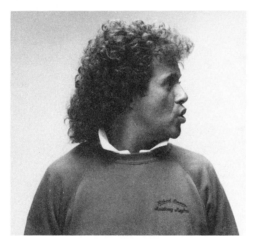

1. Turn head toward right shoulder.
2. Return to starting position.
3. Turn head toward left shoulder.
4. Return to starting position and repeat as able.

Note: This increases the neck flexibility that is often one of the first movements to become more difficult as we age.

SHOULDER AND UPPER TORSO ___
SH1   Front Arm Raises

Position: standing or sitting.
Type: Warm-up

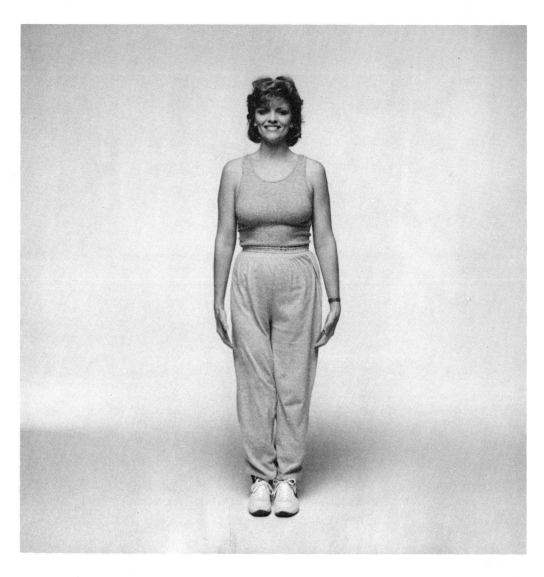

1. Drop arms alongside of body, just as Chris is doing.

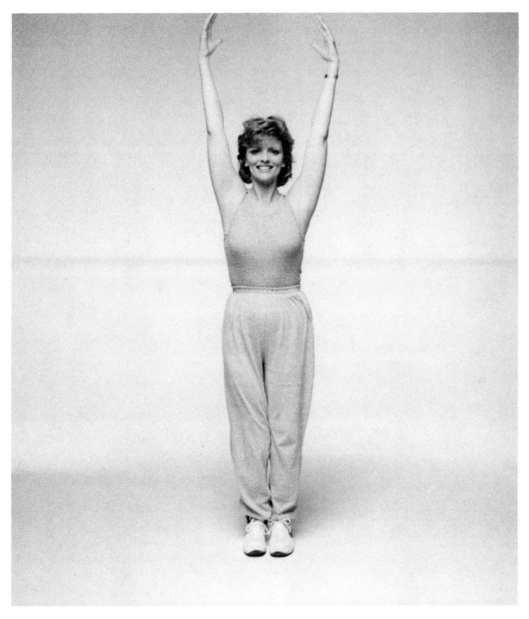

2. Keeping elbows straight, raise arms overhead.
3. Return to starting position and repeat as able.

Note: This lifting movement develops strength in the shoulder muscles and increases circulation.

SH2   Back Arm Raises

Position: standing or sitting in chair.
Type: Warm-up

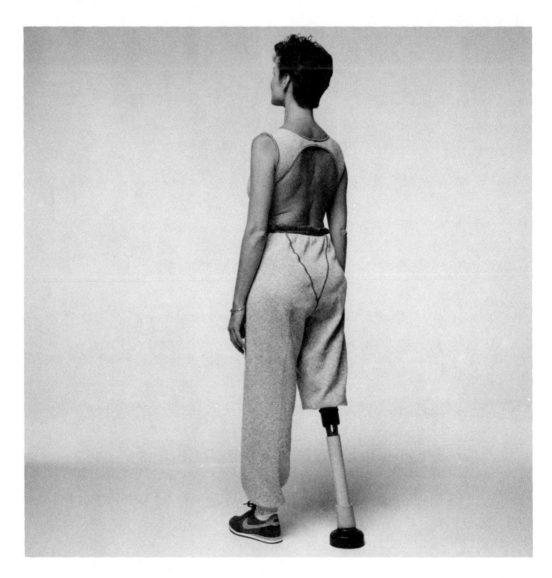

1. Drop arms alongside of body.

2. Keeping elbows straight, raise arms back as far as possible without pain.
3. Return to starting position and repeat as able.

Note: Keep trunk straight throughout exercise.

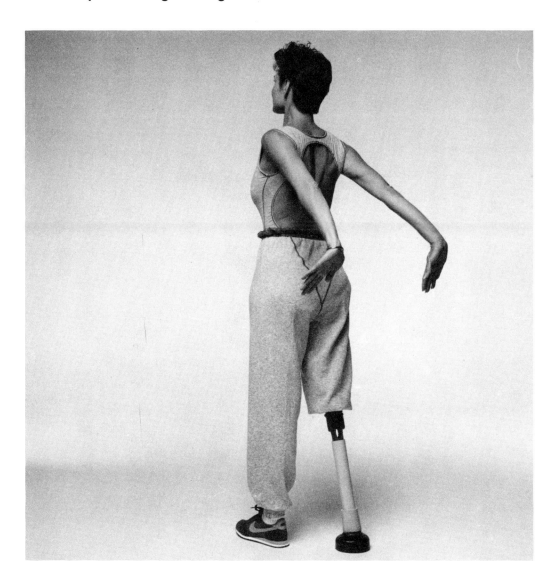

This exercise strengthens those shoulder muscles you use to move your wheelchair forward.

P.S. If you know much about prostheses for missing limbs, you've noticed that Ivy! really has a customized model!

SH3   Arm Circles

Position: standing or sitting.
Type: Warm-up

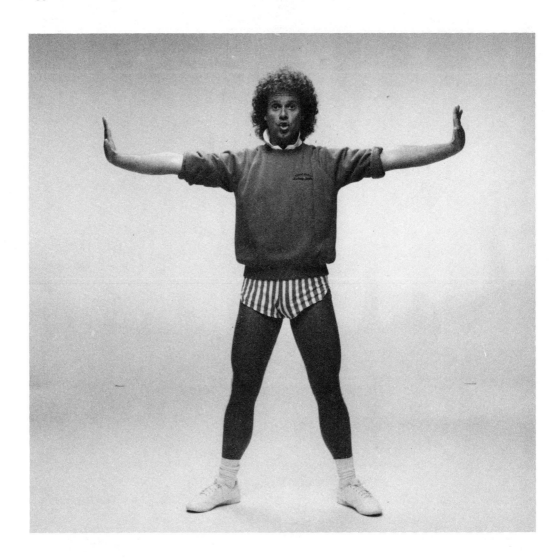

1. Straighten arms out to sides. Flex wrists.
2. Move arms forward in a large circle.
3. Reverse and circle arms backward.

Note: Rotating your arms like this helps to increase your circulation and to make you feel warmer inside.

SH4   Shoulder Shrugs

Position: standing or sitting.
Type: Warm-up

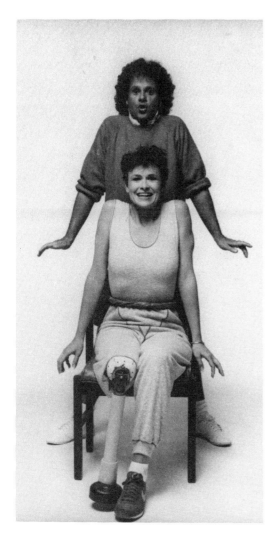 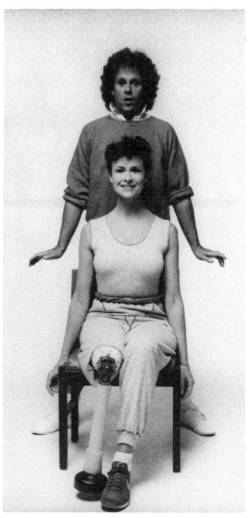

1. Shrug shoulders.
2. Drop shoulders to normal position.
3. Repeat as able.

Note: This exercise helps make your shoulders more mobile and flexible, as well as helping strengthen muscles in your neck.

SH5   Arm Presses

Position: sitting in chair with elbows bent.
Type: Isometric

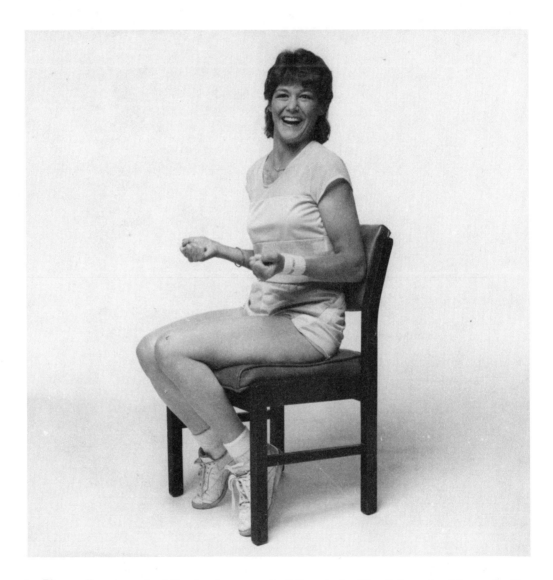

1. Place elbows against the back support of the chair. (Don't forget a big smile like Gerry's!)
2. Forcefully press elbows backward.

Note: This helps strengthen muscles necessary to lift your arms backward.

SH6   Shoulder Presses

Position: standing or sitting.
Type: Isometric

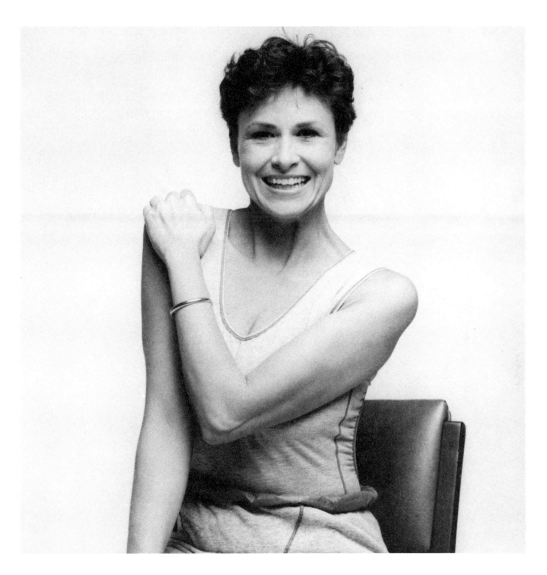

1. Place left hand on right shoulder and hold firmly.
2. Attempt to elevate shoulder against downward pressure of the hand. Hold for five seconds.
3. Alternate sides and repeat steps 1 and 2.

SH7   Side Arm Lifts

Position: standing or sitting.
Type: Isotonic

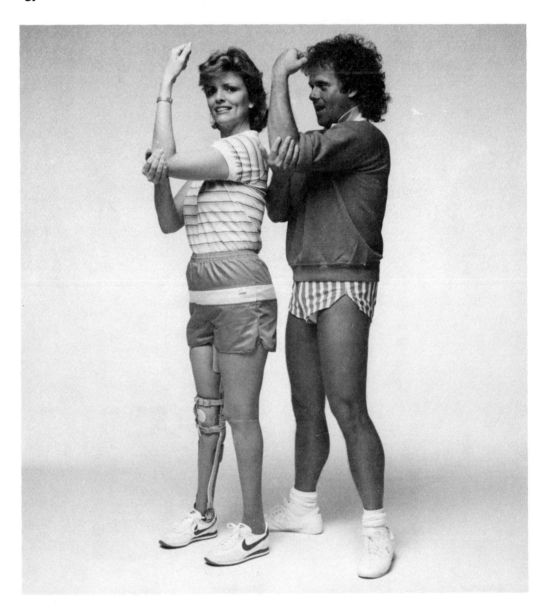

1. Bend left arm alongside of body and place right hand on left elbow.

2. Using hand to resist the movement, bring arm down as far as possible without pain.
3. Return to starting position. Repeat as able.
4. Alternate elbows and repeat as able.

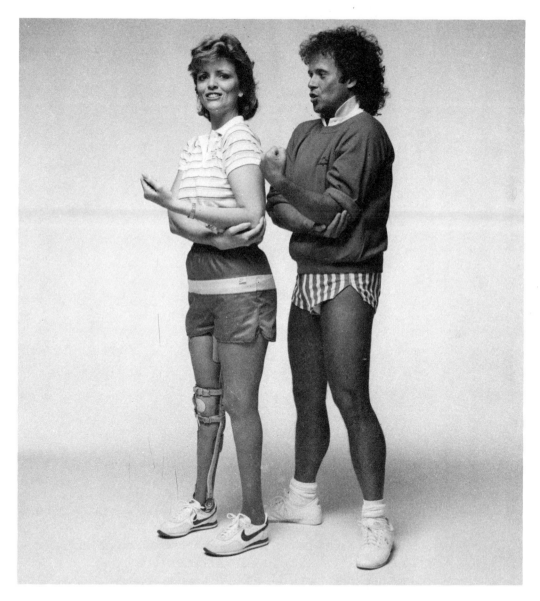

Note: This exercise will help you lift your arms to your side.

Variation: Hold weighted object in hand.

SH8   Weighted Arm Circles

Position: standing or sitting.
Type: Isotonic

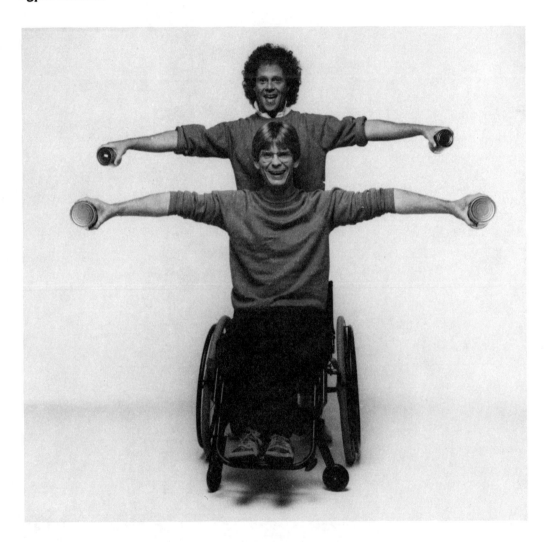

1. Holding small objects of equal weight, raise arms sideward and parallel to floor. (You'll notice that Alan and I are using cans of vegetables.)
2. Move arms forward and back in a large circle. Repeat as able.
3. Reverse direction and repeat as able.

Note: Here is an exercise that can develop overall stamina and help you in any upper-body activity.

SH9   Weighted Shoulder Shrugs

Position: standing or sitting.
Type: Isotonic

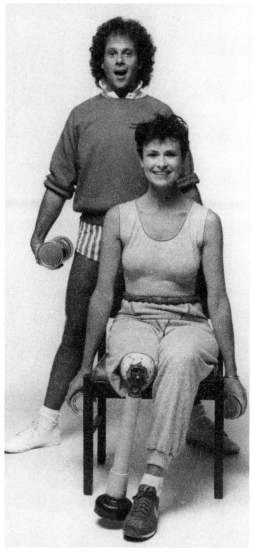 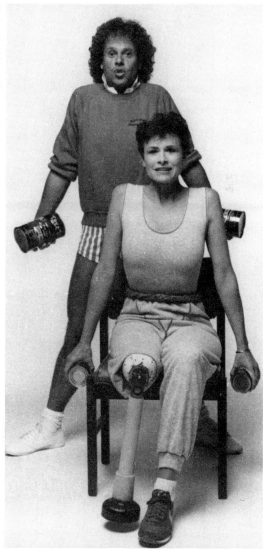

1. Holding small objects of equal weight, drop arms to sides.
2. Keeping elbows straight, shrug shoulders.
3. Return to starting position and repeat as able.

SH10 Shoulder Stretches

Position: Standing, sitting, or lying on back.
Type: Stretching/cool-down

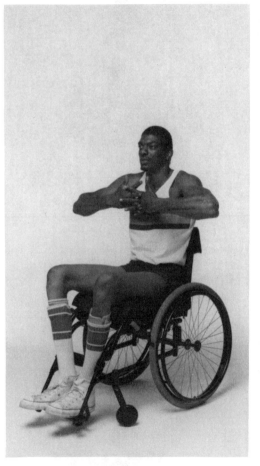 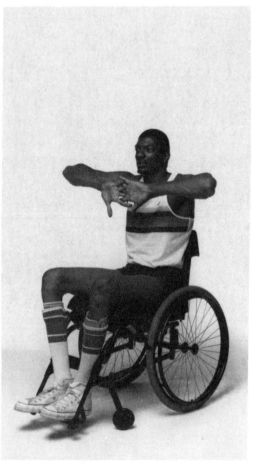

1. Interlock fingers in front of chest, the same way Bernard is doing it.
2. Turn palms out and away from chest.

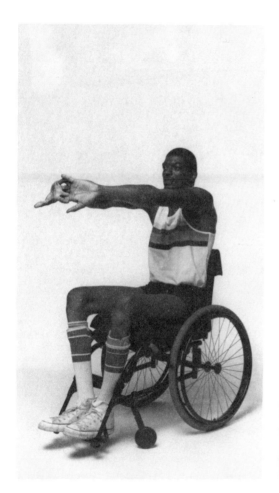 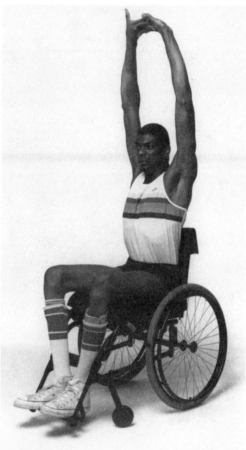

3. Slowly straighten elbows and lift arms overhead.

4. Stretch back as far as possible without pain. Hold for five to ten seconds. (This feels so good.)

Note: NEVER bounce during any stretching movement.

FOREARM
FA1   Flip-Flops

Position: standing or sitting.
Type: Warm-up

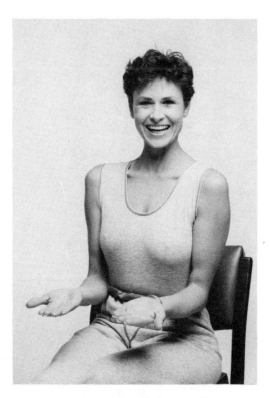

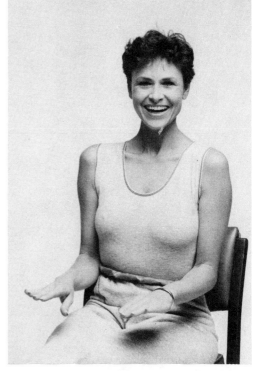

1. Hold arms in front of body with palms up and elbows touching waist.
2. Turn palms down by inwardly rotating forearms as far as possible.
3. Turn palms up by outwardly rotating forearms.
4. Repeat as able.

Note: Being able to rotate your forearms in and out like this allows you to reach and grasp things in all positions.

FA2 Can-Can

Position: sitting.
Type: Isotonic

1. Place right forearm on right thigh with palm down extending over knee.

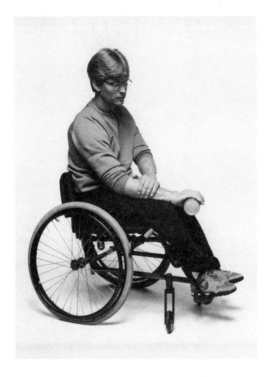

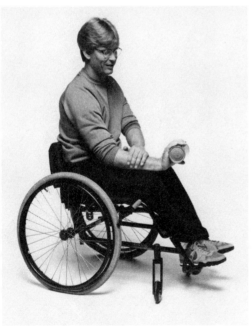

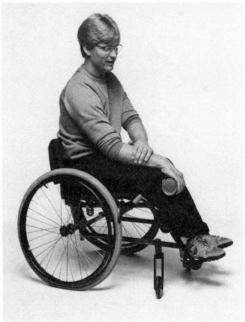

2. Grasp small weighted object and lift hand up and down. Use your left hand to stabilize the flexing forearm. Repeat as able.
3. Alternate sides and repeat as able.

ELBOW AND UPPER ARM
EUA1   Drummer

Position: standing or sitting.
Type: Warm-up

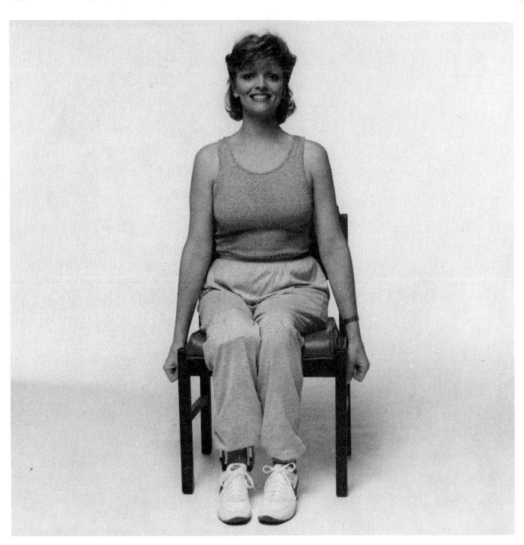

1. Drop hands at sides.

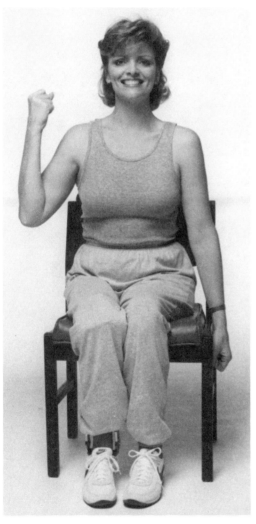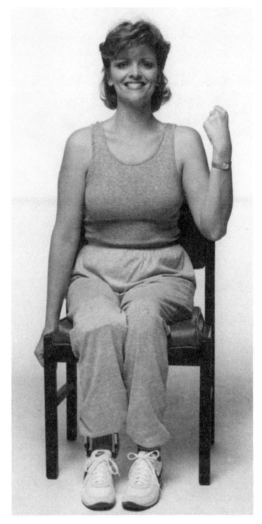

2. Alternate lifting hands toward shoulders by flexing elbows (right up, left down; left up, right down).
3. Repeat as able.

Note: This exercise strengthens muscles necessary for lifting and reaching.

Variation: Lift hands together.

EUA2   Cheerleader

Position: standing or sitting.
Type: Warm-up

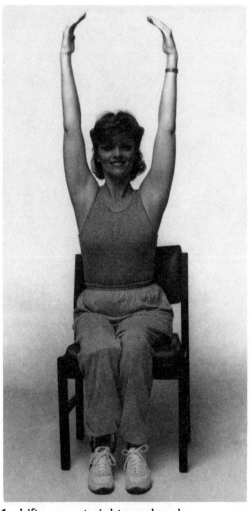 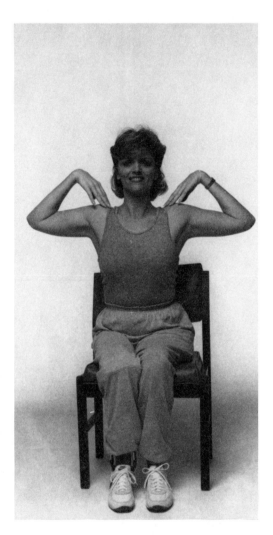

1. Lift arms straight overhead.
2. Bend elbows, allowing hands to drop toward shoulders.
3. Return to starting position and repeat as able.

Note: Keep elbows held high throughout exercise. (If you have long fingernails, don't stab your ears.)

Variation: Alternate right and left arms.

EUA3   Arm Presses

Position: sitting.
Type: Isometric

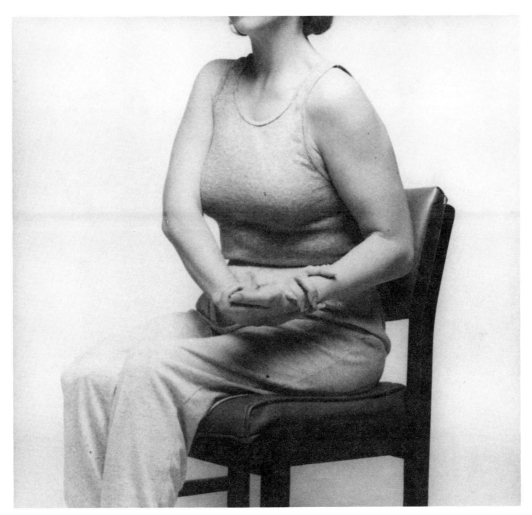

1. Place left forearm (palm up) along left thigh.
2. Grasp palm and wrist with right hand and hold firmly.
3. Press down with right hand, while trying to lift up with left forearm. Hold for five seconds.
4. Alternate sides and repeat steps 1 through 3.

Note: This exercise strengthens the biceps and triceps muscles, which are so important in lifting.

EUA4   Arm Curls

Position: standing or sitting.
Type: Isotonic

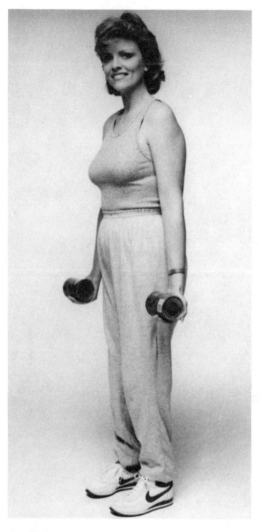 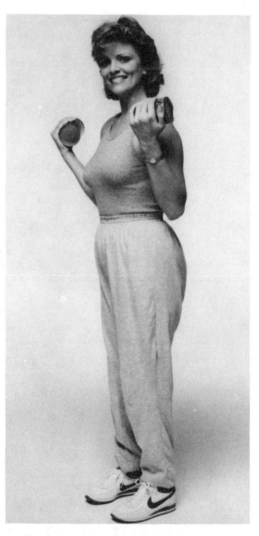

1. Hold a small weighted object in each hand and drop arms to sides (palms up).
2. Raise hands toward shoulders by bending elbows.
3. Repeat as able.

Variation: Alternate right and left hands. Repeat as able.

EUA5   Sitting Push-Ups

Position: sitting in wheelchair or chair with armrests. (If in a wheelchair, be sure wheels are locked.)

Type: Isotonic

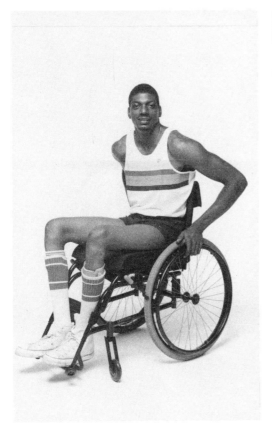 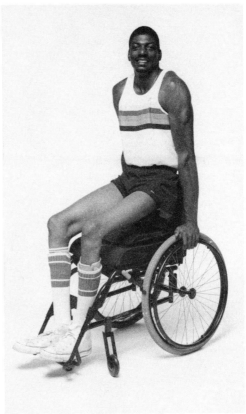

1. Grasp armrests or wheels of wheelchair (your elbows will be partially flexed).
2. Straighten elbows and lift body off chair.
3. Return to starting position and repeat as able.

Note: This exercise strengthens the triceps and back so that you can adjust your position while sitting. And being able to push up from a wheelchair is *very* important in helping you relieve pressure on your bottom.

FINGERS, WRIST, AND FOREARM
FI1   Working Hands

Position: sitting.
Type: Warm-up

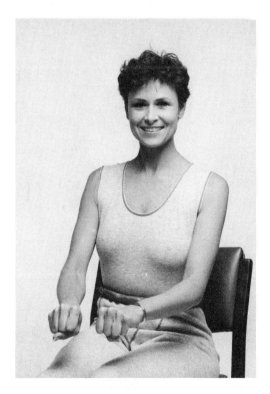

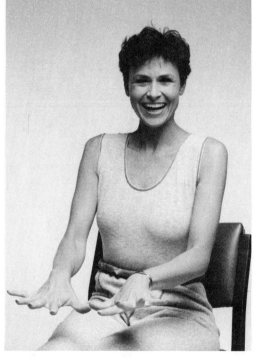

1. Place hands in lap.
2. Make fists. Squeeze.
3. Open each hand and spread fingers as far as possible.
4. Repeat as able.

FI2   Knee Grabs

Position: sitting.
Type: Isometric

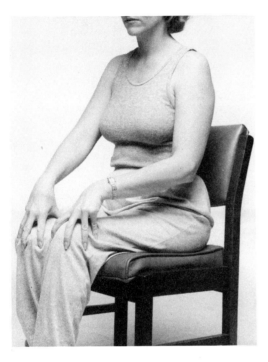

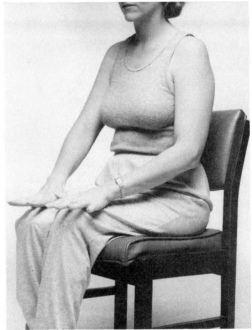

1. Place palms on knees.
2. Squeeze knees and hold for five seconds.
3. Open each hand and lift fingers as far as possible. Hold for five seconds.

Note: This exercise helps to strengthen hand muscles, which are used in all phases of daily living.

FI3   Finger Spider

Position: standing, sitting, or lying on back.
Type: Isotonic

1. Place palms and fingers together.
2. Press fingers and thumbs together as you separate palms, and pretend they are a spider climbing up a mirror.
3. Return to starting position and repeat as able.

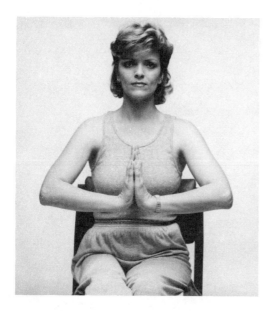

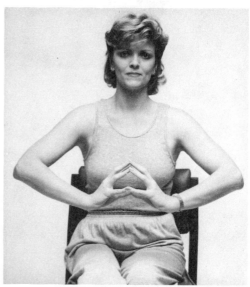

FI4 Palm Lifts

Position: sitting.
Type: Isotonic

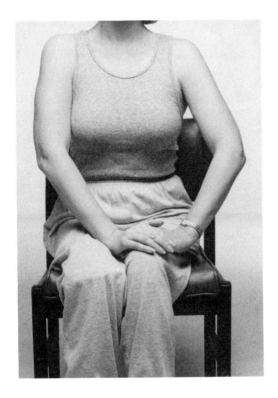

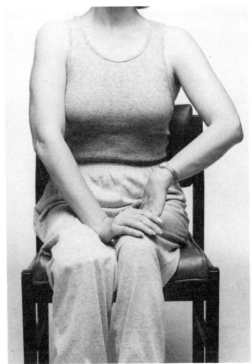

1. Place left palm (fingers down) on knee.
2. Place right palm on fingers of left hand.
3. Raise left hand against the resistance of right hand and repeat as able.
4. Alternate position and repeat as able.

FI5 Finger Stretchers

Position: standing, sitting, or lying on back.
Type: Stretching/cool-down

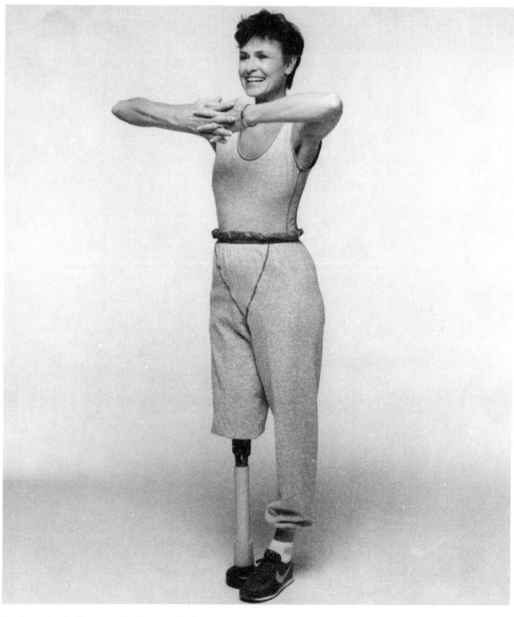

1. Interlock fingers in front of chest.
2. Slowly press hands out and extend elbows.

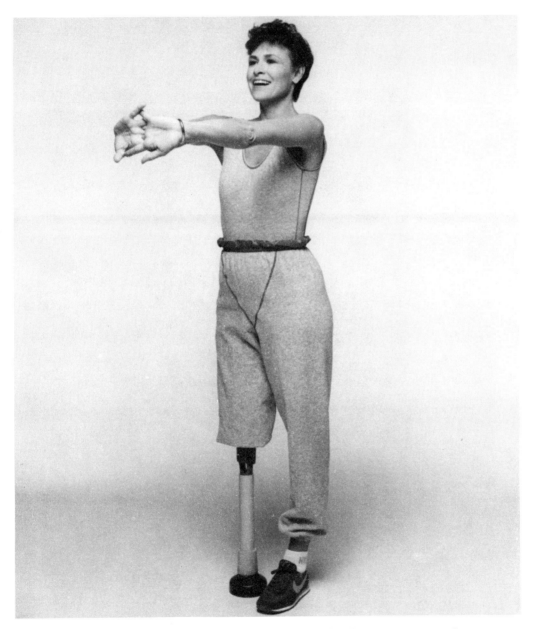

3. Stretch as far as possible without pain and hold for five to ten seconds.
4. Bring hands back to body and repeat as able.

WRIST

WR1 Waving Hands

Position: sitting.
Type: Warm-up

1. Place hands (palms up) and wrists over knees or chair armrests.
2. Curl hands toward shoulders and repeat as able.

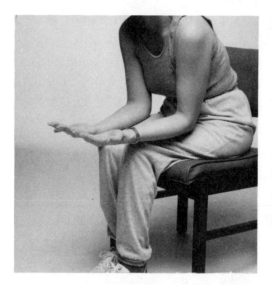 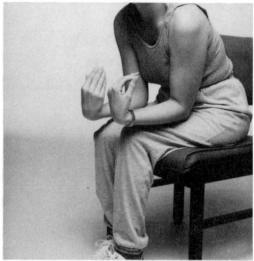

3. Now turn palms down and curl hands back toward shoulders. Repeat as able.

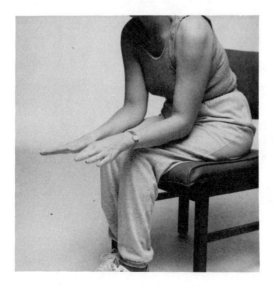 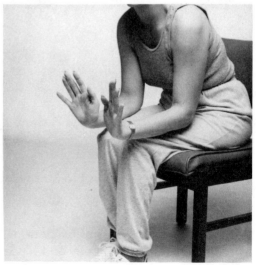

WR2   Hand Presses

Position: sitting.
Type: Isometric

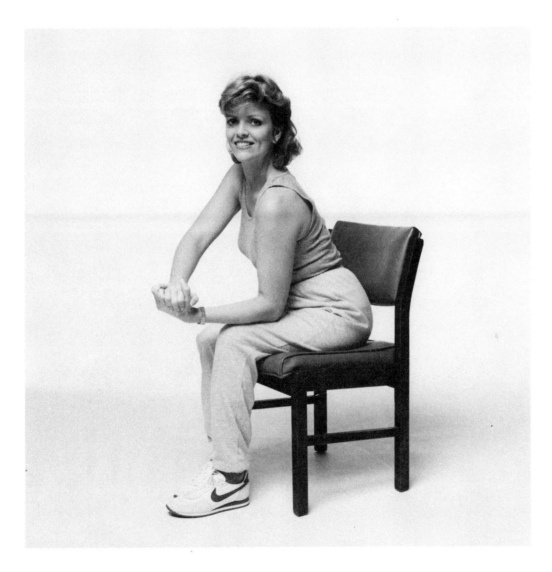

1. Place left forearm (palm up) on thigh or chair armrest.
2. Grasp left palm with right hand and hold firmly.
3. With right hand resisting movement, try to curl up left hand. Hold for five seconds.
4. Alternate hands and repeat steps 1 through 3.

WR3 Wrist Curls

Position: sitting in chair.
Type: Isotonic

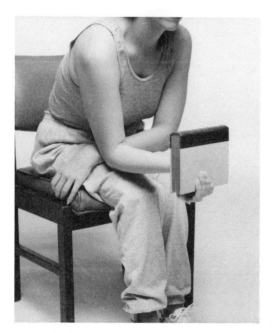

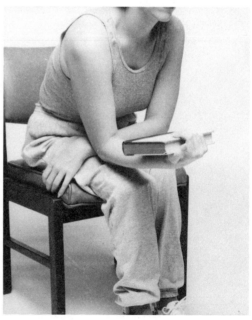

1. Hold a weighted object (like a book).
2. Position hand (palm up) over the end of a knee or chair armrest.
3. Curl wrist toward shoulder and move through full range of wrist motion or as far as possible.
4. Return to starting position and repeat as able.

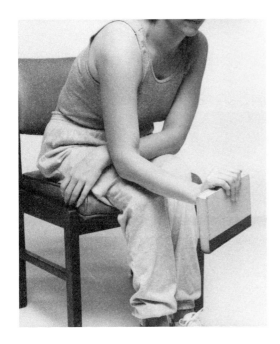

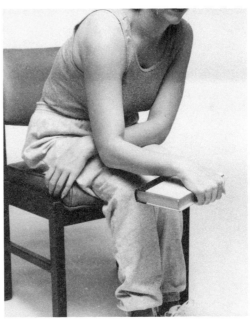

5. Now turn palm down and curl wrist down.
6. Alternate hands and repeat.

Note: Forearm should not move during exercise.

UPPER TORSO–BACK
BA1 Bent-Over Arm Raises

Position: sitting in chair.
Type: Warm-up

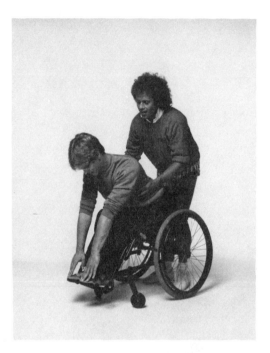

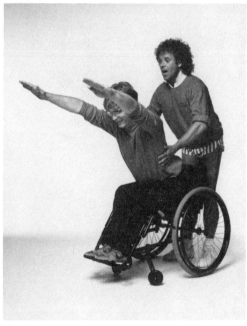

1. Bend forward at waist and drop arms to floor.
2. Elevate arms as high as possible without pain.
3. Return to starting position and repeat as able.

Note: You may want someone to help you keep your balance when doing this move.

BA2   Lift-Offs

Position: sitting.
Type: Isotonic

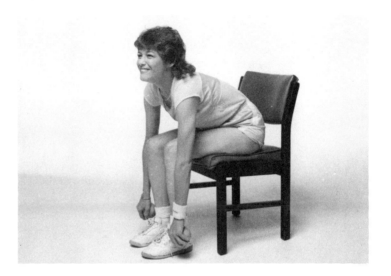

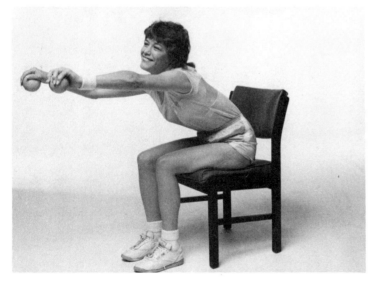

1. Holding small objects of equal weight, bend forward at waist and drop arms toward floor.
2. Lift arms upward as far as possible without pain.
3. Return to starting position and repeat as able.

BA3   Shoulder Squeeze

Position: standing or sitting.
Type: Stretching/cool-down

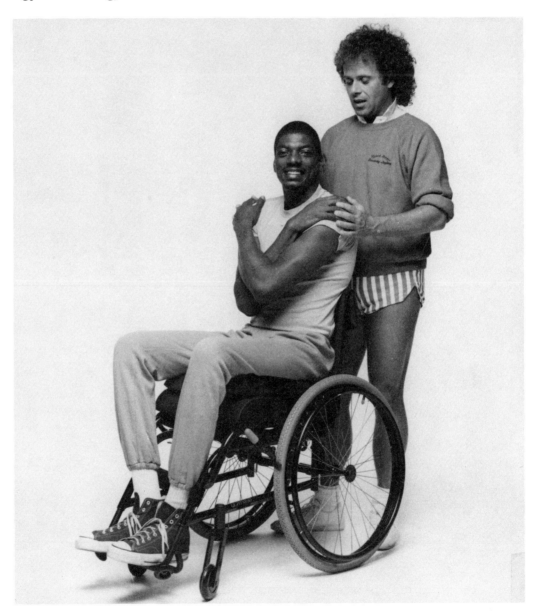

1. Place right hand on left shoulder and left hand on right shoulder.

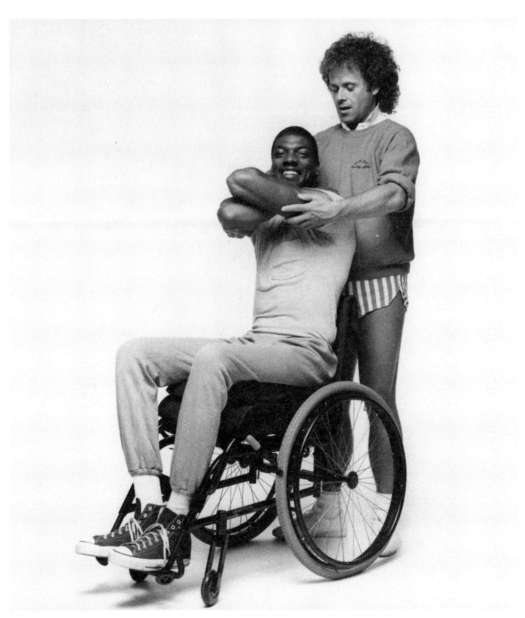

2. Lift elbows.

3. Slide hands backward, slowly tightening arms across chest, and say "hello" to your back. Hold five to ten seconds.

UPPER TORSO–CHEST
CH1   Arm Flaps

Position: lying on back with knees bent.
Type: Warm-up

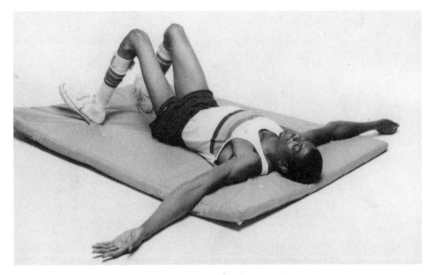

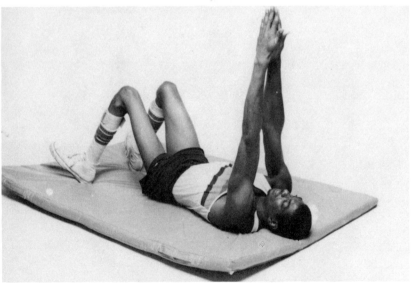

1. Extend arms sideward on floor, palms up. (You look like a big "T.")
2. Keeping elbows straight, bring arms together in front of you.
3. Return to "T" position and repeat as able.

CH2 Prayer Press

Position: standing, sitting, or lying on back with knees bent.
Type: Isometric

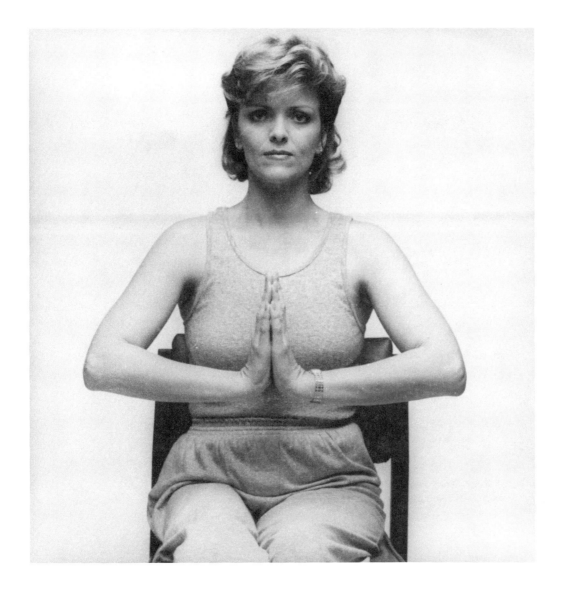

1. Place palms together in praying position.
2. Press palms together and hold for five seconds.

Note: Involves the muscles you use to reach out and pull something toward you.

CH3   Weighted Flight

Position: lying on back with knees bent.
Type: Isotonic

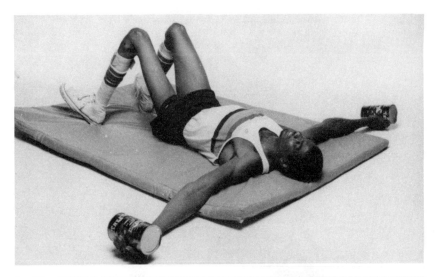

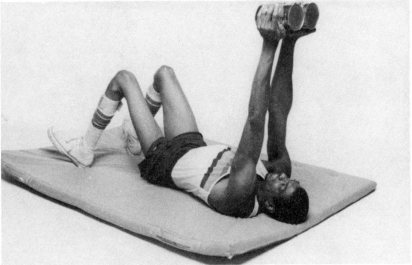

1. Hold small objects of equal weight.
2. Extend arms sideward. (You look like a big "T" again.)
3. Keeping elbows straight, bring arms together in front of you.
4. Return to "T" position and repeat as able.

CH4 Chest Stretch

Position: standing or sitting.
Type: Stretching/cool-down

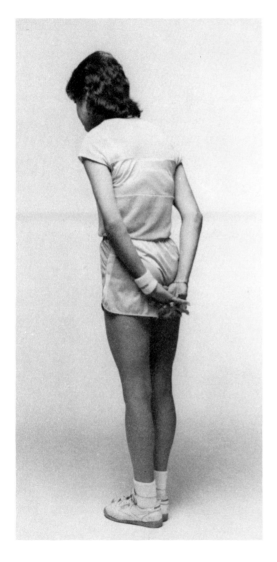 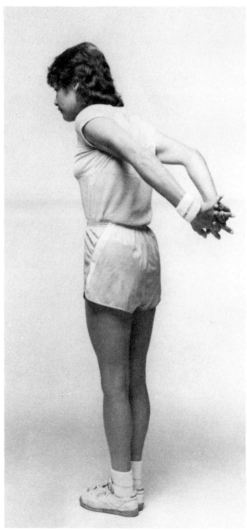

1. Clasp hands behind back.
2. Slowly push hands away and out from body while pinching shoulder blades together. Stretch as far as possible without pain. Hold for five to ten seconds.

Note: Particularly good for improving posture.

THAT VAST MIDDLE ZONE: WAIST, STOMACH, AND ABDOMINALS ___

WSA1 Back Builders

Position: sitting.
Type: Warm-up

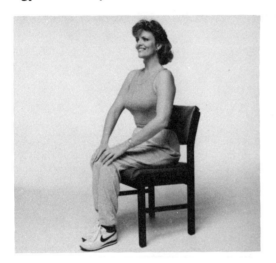
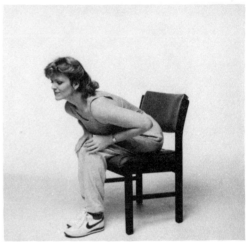

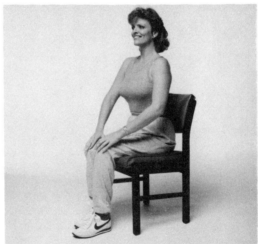

1. Place hands (palms down) on knees.
2. Bend forward at waist.
3. Keeping abdominals pulled in, return to starting position and repeat as able.

Note: Avoid pushing up with your hands—unless absolutely necessary.

WSA2   Tummy Tuckers

Position: lying on back, knees bent, feet flat.
Type: Warm-up

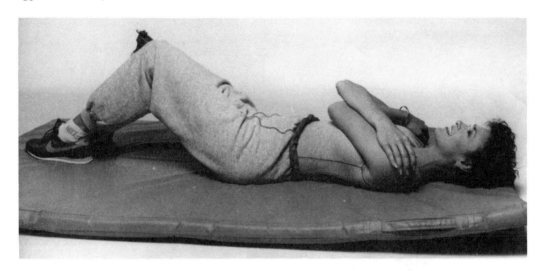

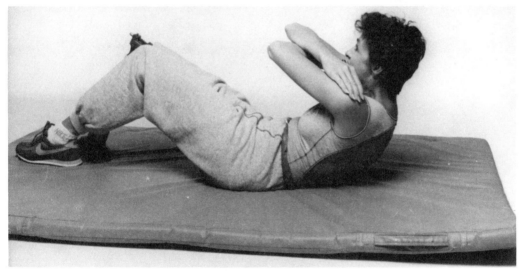

1. Place arms across chest, each hand on opposite shoulder. Tighten stomach muscles.
2. In one smooth movement, lift head and shoulders. Hold for five to ten seconds.
3. Return to starting position and repeat as able.

Note: If this is too difficult, an easier variation is to lie flat and alternate tightening and releasing your stomach muscles.

WSA3　Side Trimmers

Position: standing or sitting.
Type: Warm-up

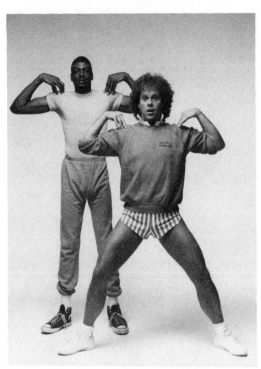

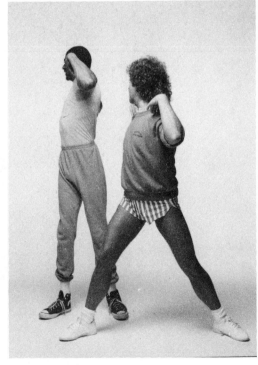

1. Lift elbows to shoulder level, hands on shoulders.
2. Rotate trunk by slowly twisting head, shoulders, and arms from side to side.

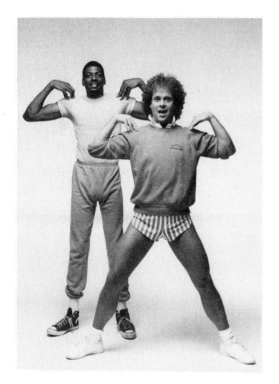

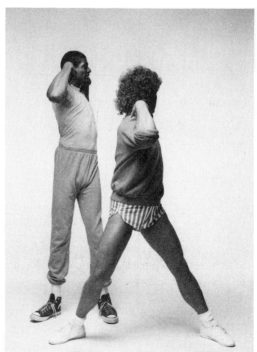

Note: Hold hips still and try to look to the wall behind you.

WSA4 Trunk Twist-Press

Position: sitting.
Type: Isometric

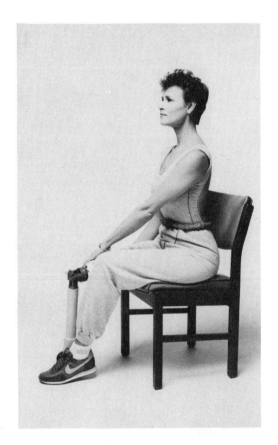
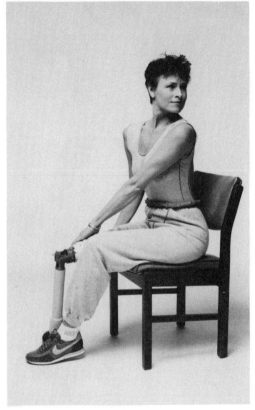

1. Place left hand on right thigh and lock elbow.
2. Using left arm to resist movement, rotate trunk toward your left side. Hold for five seconds.
3. Alternate sides and repeat as able.

Note: This exercise helps develop the lateral muscles that turn and twist the body, and which are necessary for walking.

WSA5   Curl-Ups

Position: lying flat on back or with legs on a chair, as Alan demonstrates.
Type: Isotonic

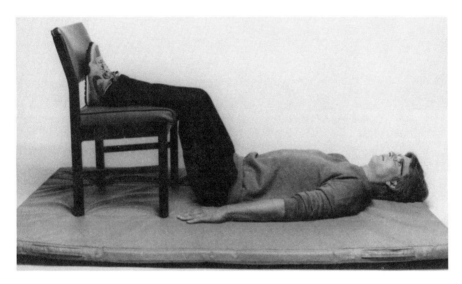

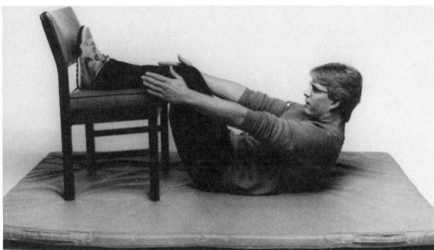

1. Place arms at sides, palms down.
2. Lift head and shoulders off surface and reach for knees.
3. Return to starting position and repeat as able.

Note: Even though Alan doesn't have one, beer bellies are helped by this exercise.

WSA6   Prone Lifts

Position: lying on stomach.
Type: Isotonic

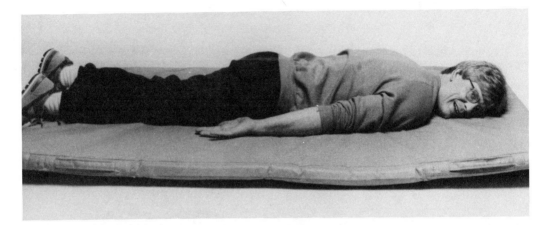

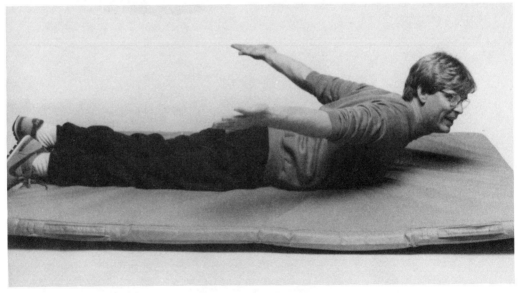

1. Place arms (palms up) alongside of body.
2. Lift head, chest and arms. Try to pinch your shoulder blades together.
3. Return to starting position and repeat as able.

Note: This is good for posture (especially if you've been sitting all day).

WSA7   Side Stretchers

Position: standing or sitting. (If sitting, hold on to one side of the chair.)
Type: Stretching/cool-down

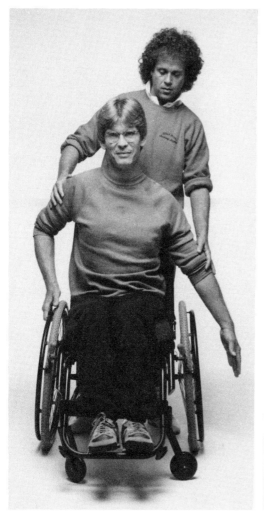 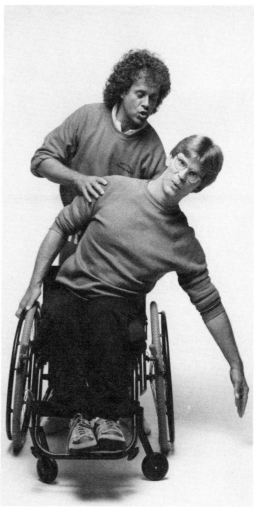

1. Drop arms to sides.
2. Bending sideward, stretch left hand toward floor. Return to starting position and repeat as able.
3. Alternate sides and repeat as able.

Caution: If you have trouble maintaining your balance during this exercise, ask someone to help.

HIPS AND BUTTOCKS
HB1 Rear Leg Raises

Position: standing, holding on to something solid (like a piece of furniture).
Type: Warm-up

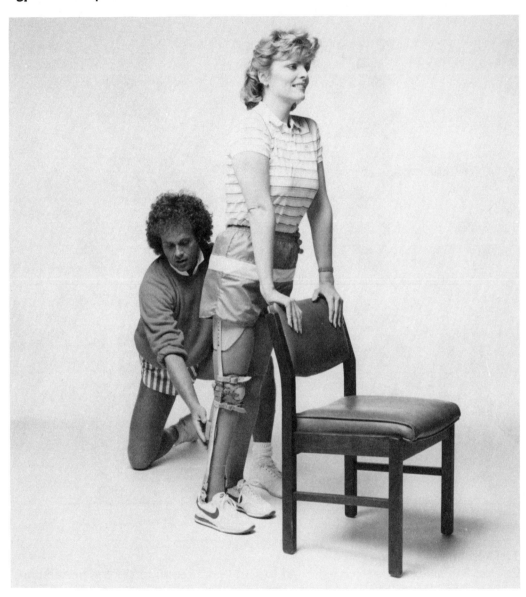

1. Keeping knee straight, lift right leg behind body. Keep trunk slightly forward, and hold hips still.
2. Return to starting position and repeat as able.
3. Alternate legs and repeat as able.

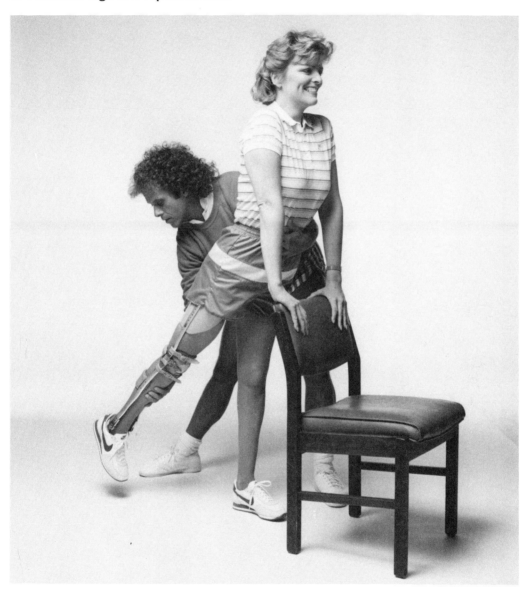

Note: Be sure to keep stomach muscles tight, and do not arch your lower back during exercise. It's okay for someone to gently help until you can do this on your own.

Leg muscles used in this exercise are essential for standing and walking.

HB2   Show Biz

Position: lying on back, knees bent.
Type: Warm-up

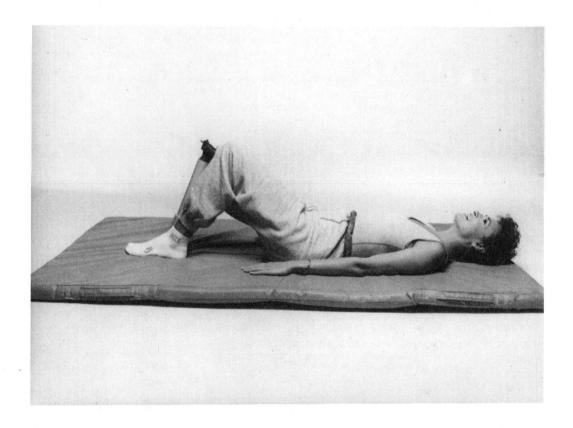

1. Lift left leg off floor, bringing knee toward chest.

2. Using both hands, firmly grasp back of knee.
3. Attempt to pull knee to chest.
4. Extend leg and hold for five seconds. Return to starting position and repeat as able.
5. Alternate sides and repeat as able.

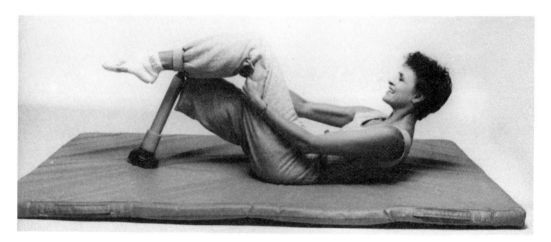

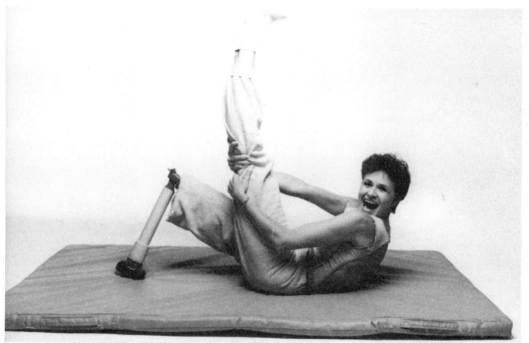

Note: Helps the muscles you use when you stand up from a chair or climb stairs.
    P.S. Don't be discouraged if you can't get the same extension as Ivy! She's been practicing.

HB3   Bridging

Position: lying on back, knees bent, hands at sides.
Type: Isotonic

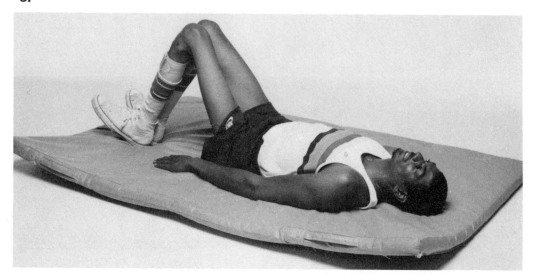

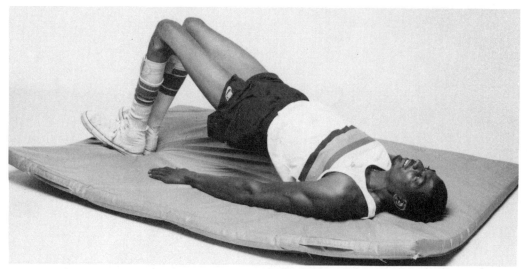

1. Keeping your feet and knees together, lift your hips off the floor, mat, or bed. (Remember, your hips are the weight you are lifting.)
2. Slowly lower yourself to starting position and repeat as able.

Note: Strengthens most of the back of the body.

HB4   Stiff Leg Lifts

Position: lying on stomach.
Type: Isotonic

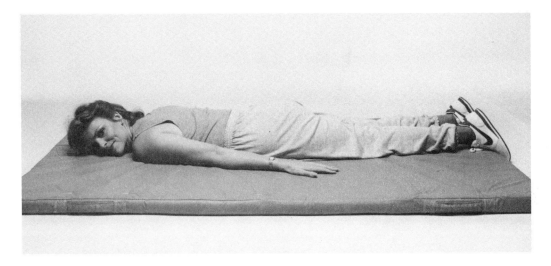

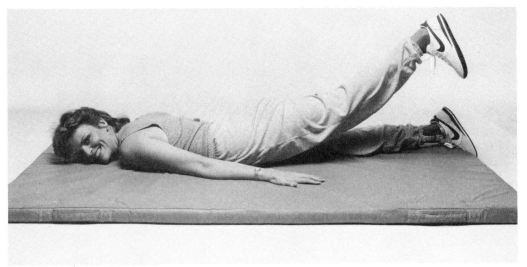

1. Place arms (palms down) alongside of body.
2. Lock left knee and lift leg as high as possible.
3. Slowly lower leg. Repeat as able.
4. Alternate sides and repeat as able.

Note: Added resistance can be achieved by attaching a weighted object to your foot. (I just know you'll come up with something imaginative!)

HB5   Back Leg Stretches

Position: lying on back with knees bent.
Type: Stretching/cool-down

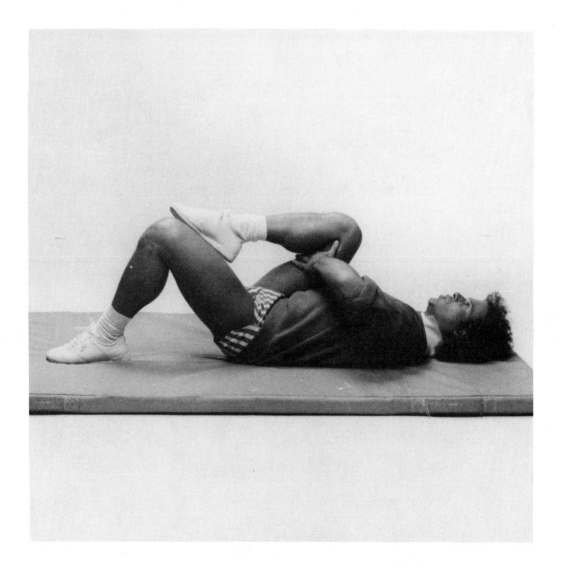

1. Bring right knee toward chest.

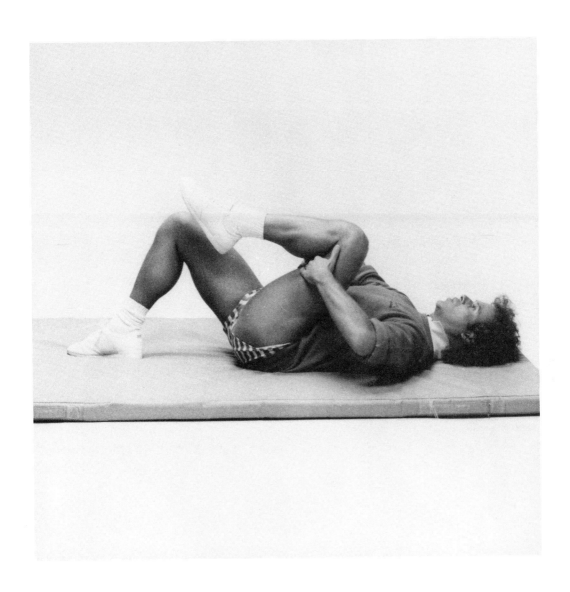

2. With both hands, grasp behind knee and slowly pull knee as close to chest as possible. Stop when you feel any discomfort. Hold for five to ten seconds.
3. Alternate legs and repeat as able.

HB6   Side Lifts

Position: lying on side, legs straight. (If you feel any discomfort, you can bend lower leg.)
Type: Warm-up

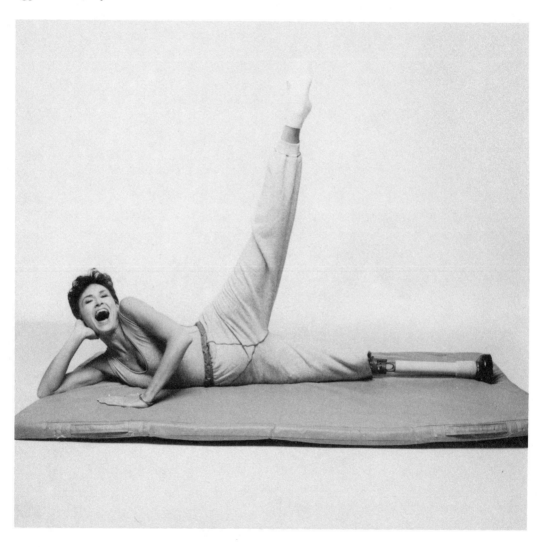

1. Lift top leg as high as possible.

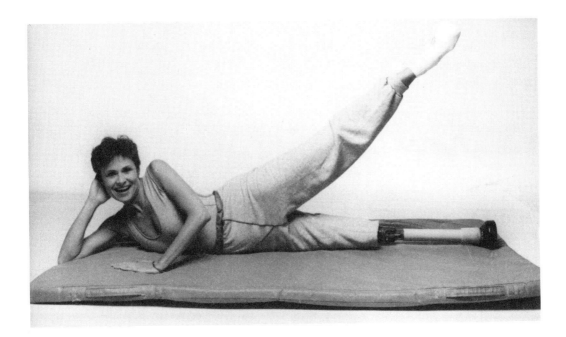

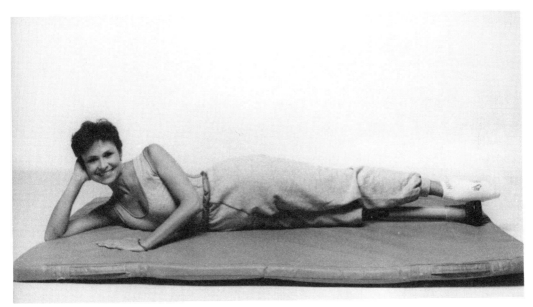

2. Slowly lower leg. Repeat as able.
3. Alternate sides and repeat as able.

Note: The muscles used in this set of exercises are important for walking, and they also are the ones that soften up and hang on your legs like "saddlebags."
    P.S. Once again, Ivy's been practicing!

HB7   Outside Hip Press

Position: sitting.
Type: Isometric

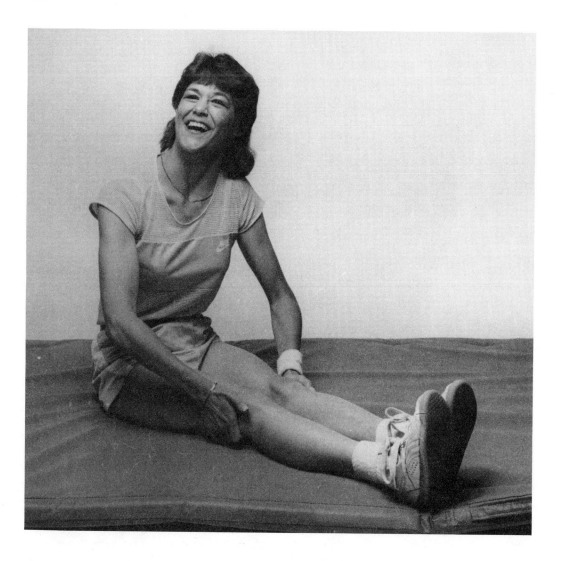

1. Place hands on outsides of knees and hold firmly.
2. Using hands to resist movement, try to force knees apart. Hold for five seconds.

Note: Gerry doesn't have them, but saddlebags can be stamped out with this exercise!!

HB8   Moving Hip Press

Position: sitting on floor, knees bent, or sitting in chair, knees together.
Type: Isotonic

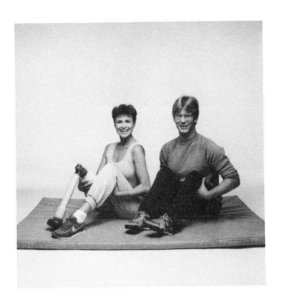

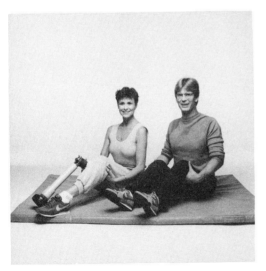

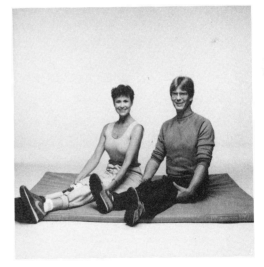

1. Place hands behind knees and hold firmly.
2. Using hands to provide some resistance, move legs through full range of outward motion.

HB9 Side Leg Stretches

Position: sitting on flat surface.
Type: Stretching/cool-down

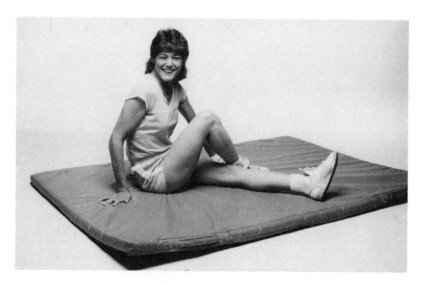

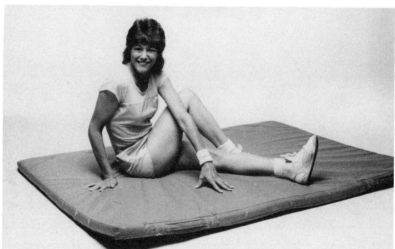

1. Keeping left leg straight, cross right leg over left knee.
2. Support body with right arm. (If you omit this step, you'll fall right over.)
3. Place left arm on outside of right leg.
4. Now slowly press your right leg toward left arm as far as you can without discomfort. Hold for five to ten seconds. Repeat as able.
5. Alternate sides and repeat as able.

HB10 Frog Flaps

Position: lying on back, knees bent.
Type: Warm-up

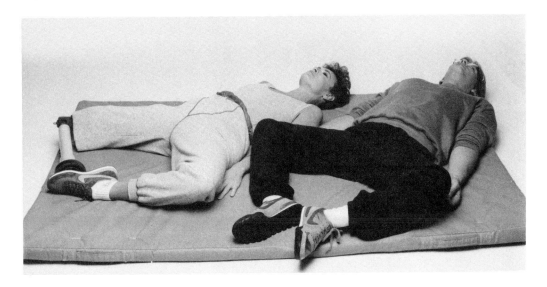

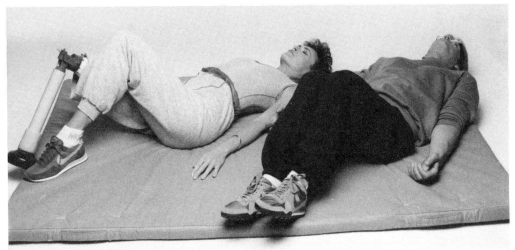

1. Bring soles of feet together, and spread knees apart as far as possible without pain.
2. Now bring knees together and repeat as able.

HB11   Leg Squeeze

Position: sitting on flat surface, legs spread, or sitting in chair with knees apart.
Type: Isometric

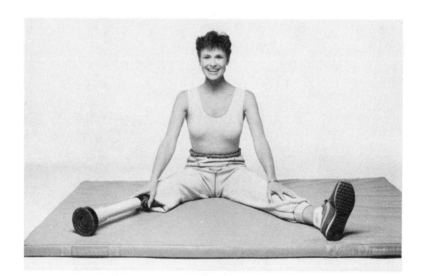

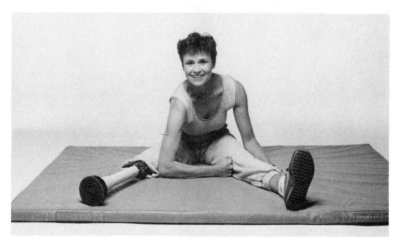

1. Horizontally wedge right forearm between knees.
2. Try to squeeze knees together. Hold for five seconds.

Note: The fist of your hand and the back of your elbow should be pressing against the insides of your knees.

HB12   Inside Leg Stretch

Position: sitting on flat surface, knees bent.
Type: Stretching/cool-down

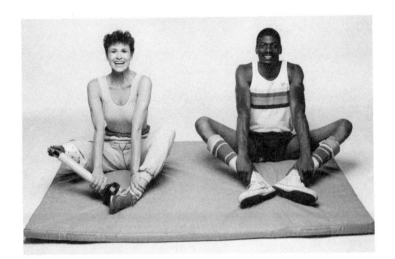

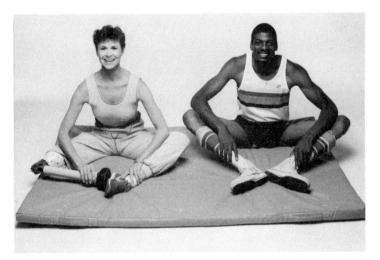

1. Bring feet together, and spread knees as far as possible without pain.
2. Grasp ankles and slowly lean forward as you press forearms down against legs.
3. Push as far down as possible without pain. Hold for five to ten seconds. Do not bounce!

Note: Many people (particularly those with spastic muscles) have tightness in the muscles worked here.

HB13 Front Leg Raises

Position: sitting or lying on back with knees bent.
Type: Warm-up

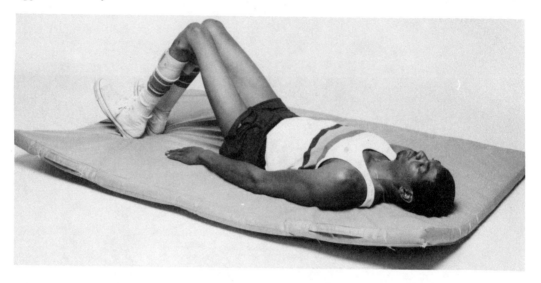

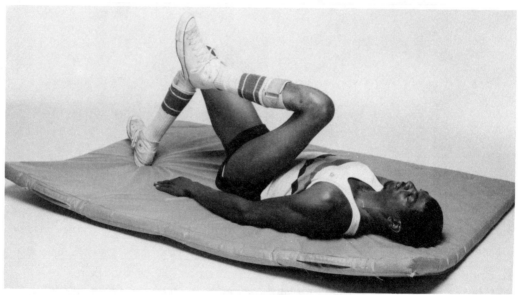

1. Bring right knee to chest.
2. Return to starting position and repeat as able.
3. Alternate knees and repeat as able.

HB14   Front Leg Presses

Position: sitting in chair or lying on back with knees bent.
Type: Isometric

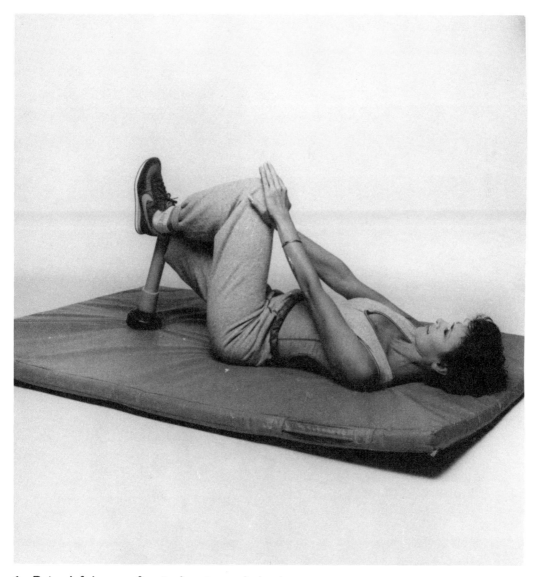

1. Raise left knee a few inches toward chest.
2. Place both hands just above the knee and hold firmly.
3. Using hands to resist movement, attempt to lift knee toward chest. Hold for five seconds.
4. Alternate knees and repeat steps 1 through 3.

HB15   Moving Leg Presses

Position: sitting in chair or lying on back with knees bent.
Type: Isotonic

1. Place hands on both knees.

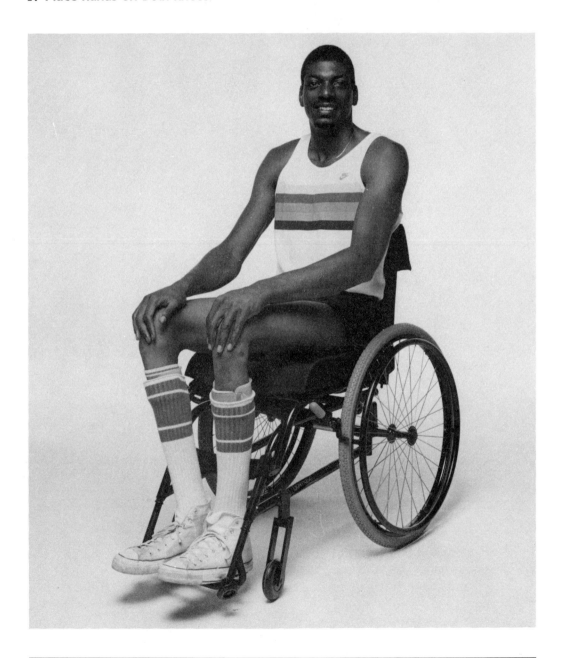

2. Using left hand to provide resistance, raise left knee a few inches toward chest.
3. Return to starting position and repeat as able.
4. Alternate knees and repeat as able.

Variation: Alternate knees in succession as if you were in a marching band.

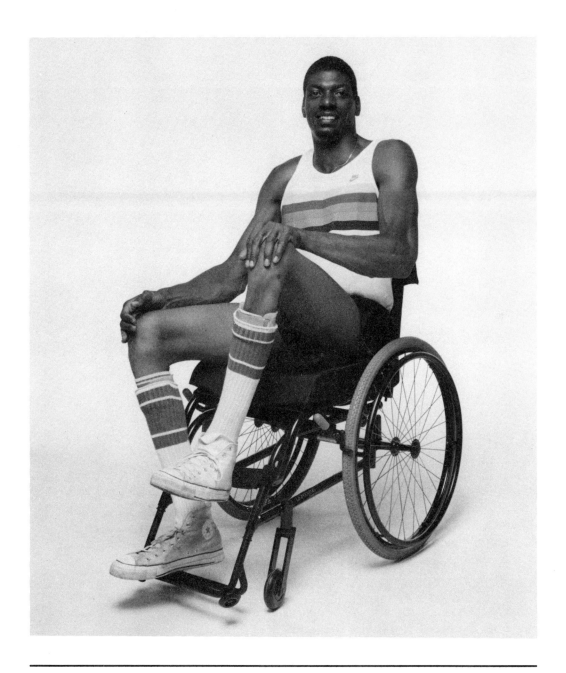

THIGHS AND KNEES
TK1   Kick Outs

Position: sitting in chair.
Type: Warm-up

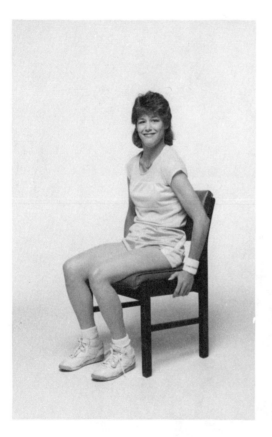 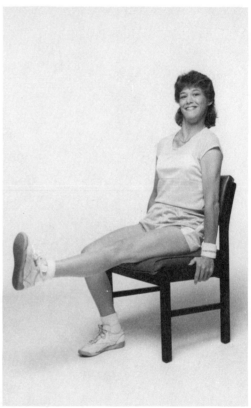

1. Extend left leg forward until it is parallel to the floor.
2. Return to starting position and repeat as able.
3. Alternate legs and repeat as able.

Note: The muscles worked in this set of exercises are important for standing and walking. You've heard that you should lift with your legs and not your back; well, these are the powerful muscles that do it.

TK2   Kick Press

Position: sitting in chair.
Type: Isometric

1. Place left ankle on top of right ankle.
2. Using left leg to resist movement, try to straighten right leg. Hold for five seconds.
3. Alternate legs and repeat steps 1 and 2.

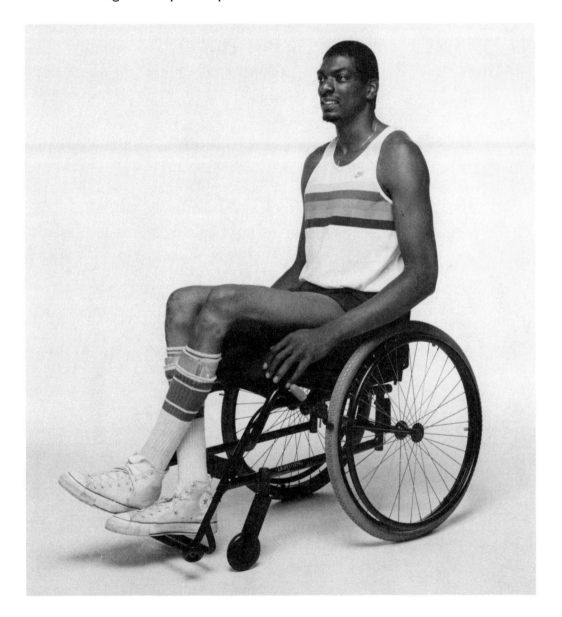

TK3   Moving Kick Presses

Position: sitting.
Type: Isotonic

1. Place right ankle on top of left ankle.

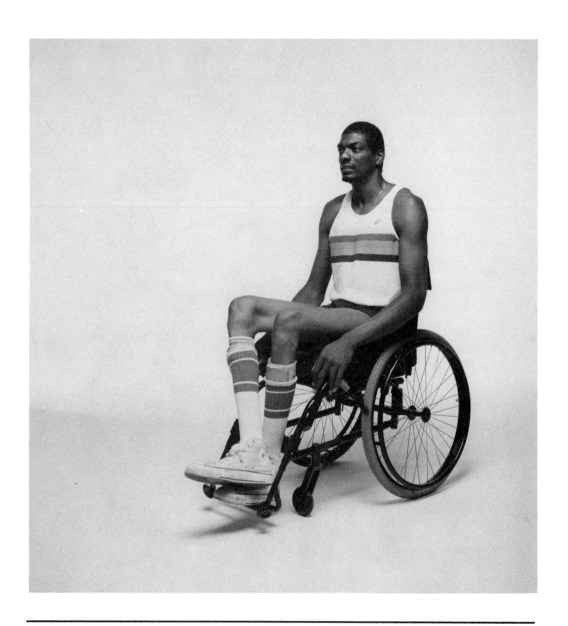

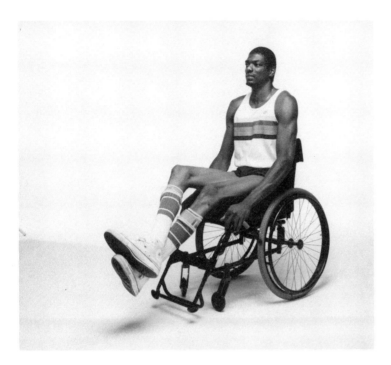

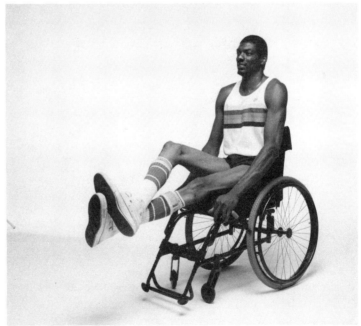

2. Using right leg to provide some resistance, move left leg through its full range of motion. Return to starting position and repeat as able.

3. Alternate legs and repeat as able.

TK4   Kick Backs

Position: lying on stomach, upper body propped up on elbows.
Type: Warm-up

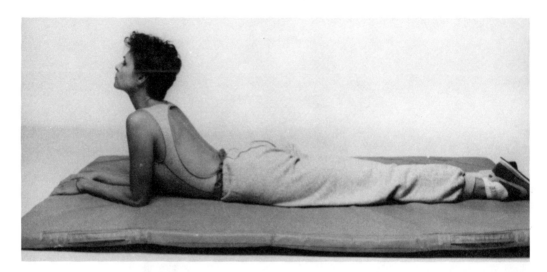

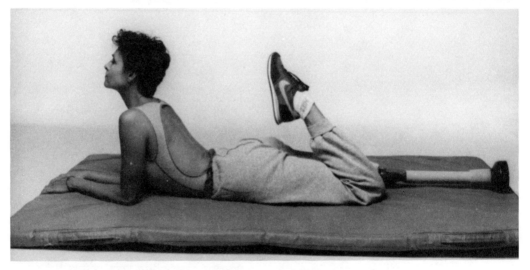

1. Bending left knee, bring heel as close to buttocks as possible.
2. Return to starting position and repeat as able.
3. Alternate legs and repeat as able.

Note: You need these muscles to work the hip and extend the knee when you walk. They're major muscles used in running, biking, swimming, and many other athletic movements.

TK5 Kick Back Presses

Position: lying on stomach, upper body propped up on elbows.
Type: Isometric

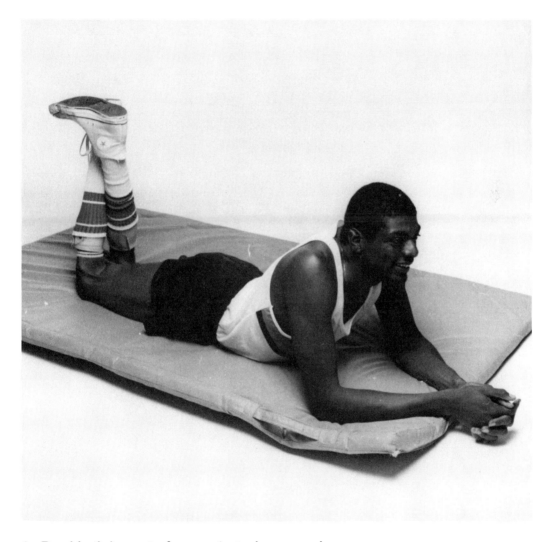

1. Bend both knees to form a ninety-degree angle.
2. Place the left ankle behind the right ankle.
3. Using left leg to resist the movement, try to flex right leg. Hold for five seconds.
4. Alternate legs and repeat steps 1 through 3.

TK6   Kick Back Lifts

Position: lying on stomach, upper body propped up on elbows.
Type: Isotonic

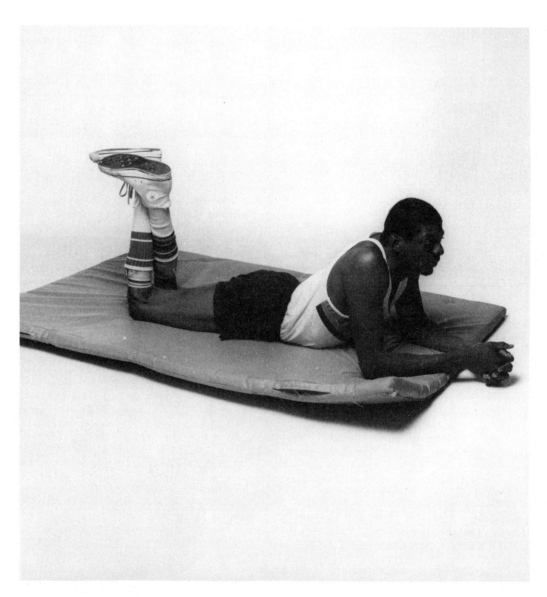

1. Place the top of left foot over the heel of right foot.
2. Using left leg to provide some resistance, move right knee through its full range of motion. Repeat as able.
3. Alternate legs and repeat as able.

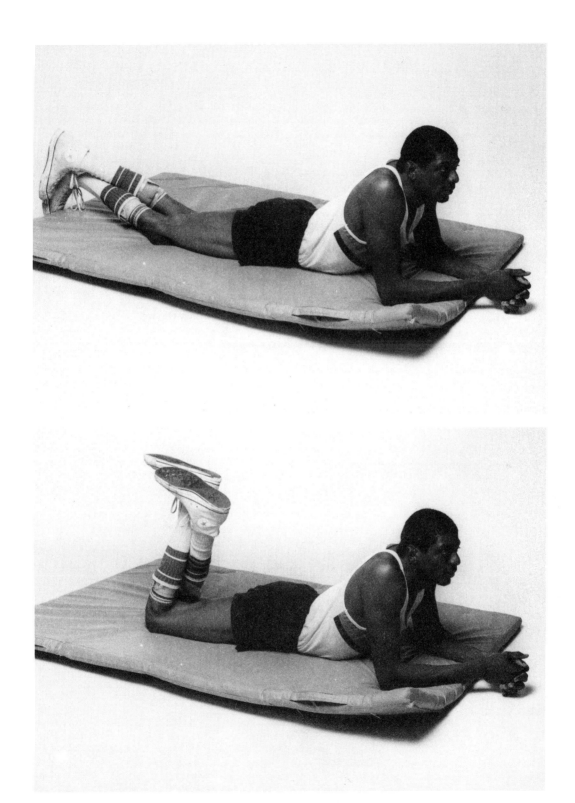

TK7 Wheelchair Walk

Position: sitting in wheelchair.
Type: Isotonic

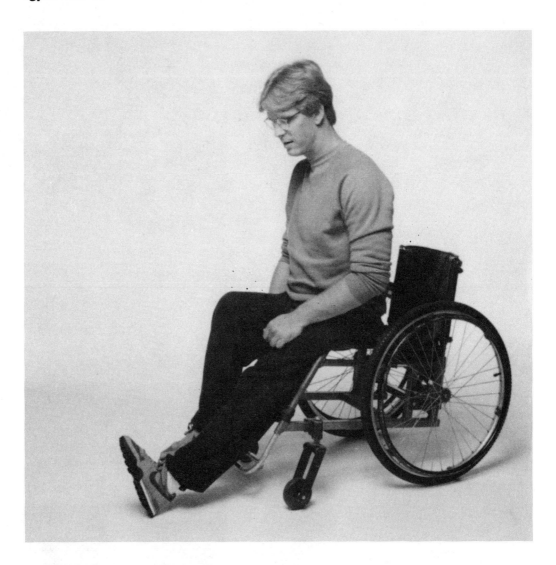

1. Release brake on wheelchair.
2. Move left leg forward and dig heel into floor.

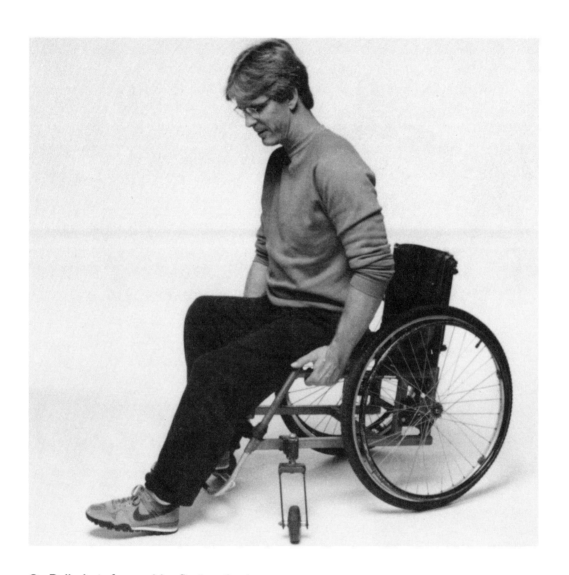

3. Pull chair forward by flexing the knee.
4. Repeat as able.

Variation: This exercise can also be done with both legs at a time or by alternating legs.
   Make it into a race—and keep going until you decide that you've won!

TK8   Back Thigh Stretchers

Position: sitting, legs straight. (If in a wheelchair, you can prop leg up as shown.)
Type: Stretching/cool-down

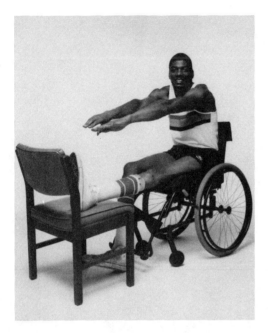

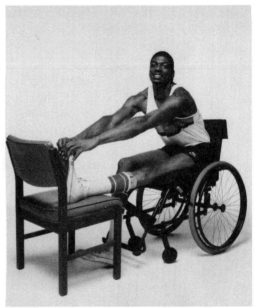

1. Slowly bend forward at waist and reach for your left foot.
2. Continue movement until you feel a comfortable stretching in the back of knee and thigh. Hold for five to ten seconds.
3. Return to starting position and repeat as able.

Note: Make certain that your chest is up, your abdominals are pulled in, and your back is straight. Be careful not to bounce!

*FOOT, ANKLE, AND LOWER LEG*___

FAL1   Foot Flappers

Position: sitting in chair or on side of bed, shoes off.
Type: Warm-up

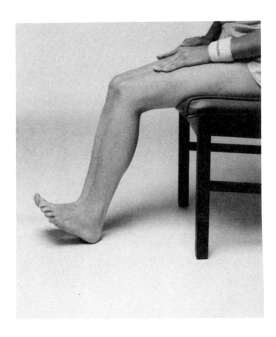

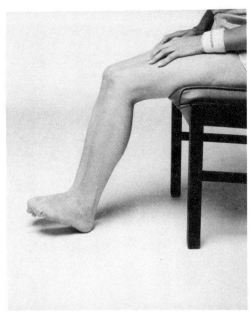

1. Push feet forward until just the heels touch the floor.
2. Curl toes away from body.
3. Return to starting position and move toes back toward body.
4. Repeat as able.

FAL2   Foot Winders

Position: sitting in chair.
Type: Warm-up

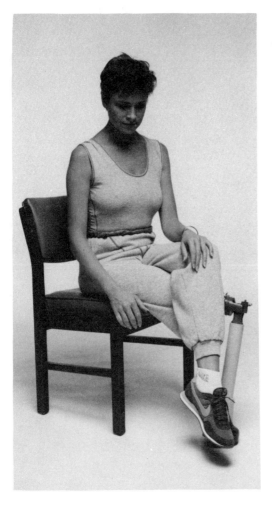 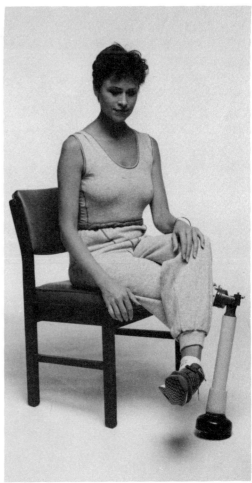

1. Cross left leg over right knee.
2. Circle left foot, first to the right and then to the left. Repeat as able.
3. Alternate legs and repeat as able.

Note: For strengthening the muscles along the side of your ankle.

FAL3 High Heels

Position: standing, holding on to a solid object (back of chair, heavy furniture, or countertop).
Type: Isometric

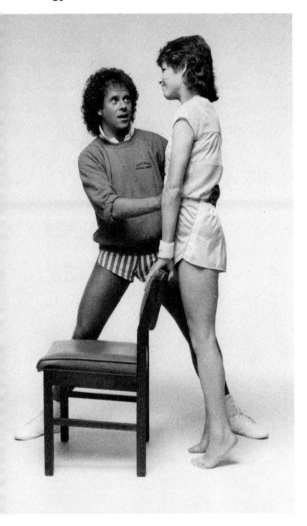
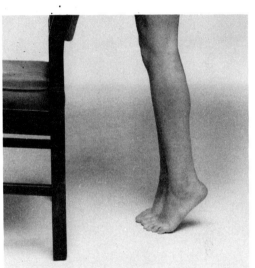

1. Stand up on toes. Hold for five to ten seconds.
2. Return to starting position.

Note: Helps give shape and tone to the calf muscles.

This exercise can become isotonic by moving up and down on toes for as many repetitions as able. (The weight you would be moving then would be your own body.)

FAL4   Foot Presses

Position: sitting in chair, shoes off.
Type: Isometric

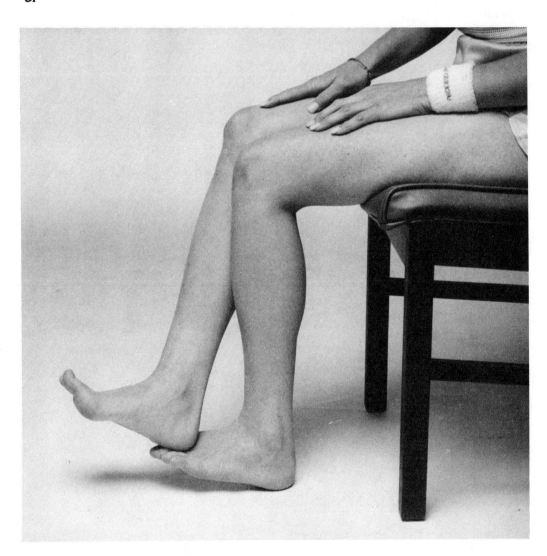

1. Press right foot down on the top of left foot. (Stay near the toes.)
2. Using right foot to resist movement, raise left foot, heel remaining on floor. Hold for five seconds. Return to starting position and repeat as able.
3. Alternate feet and repeat steps 1 and 2.

FAL5 Toe Pick-Ups

Position: sitting, shoes off.
Type: Isotonic

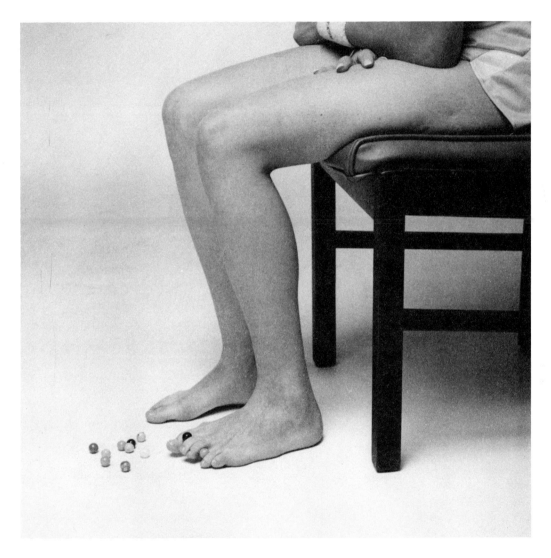

1. Pick up small objects (marbles, pencils, paper wads, etc.) with the toes of your left foot.
2. Bring left foot up and drop objects in (or near) your right hand. Repeat as able.
3. Alternate sides and repeat as able.

Note: Very good for weak arches. It takes practice, but you can do it!

FAL6   Towel Pull

Position: sitting in chair or on side of bed, shoes off.
Type: Isotonic

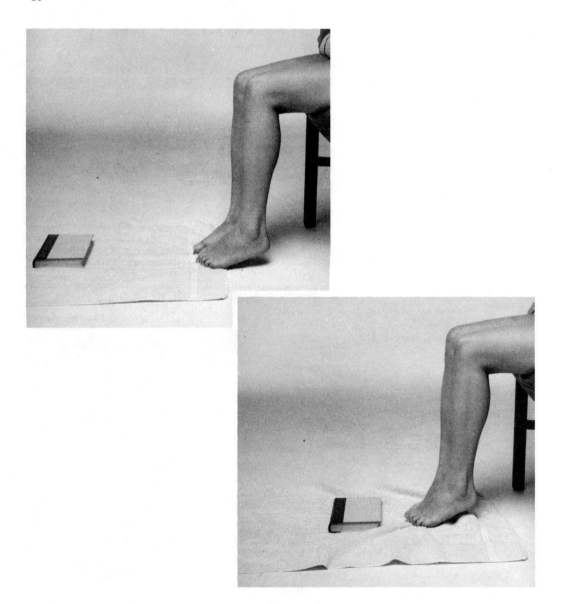

1. Place the end of a towel under your feet. At the opposite end, place a weighted object, like a book.
2. Using the curling action of your toes, pull the book toward you.

FAL7 Wall Push-Ups

Position: standing, facing wall at arm's distance.
Type: Stretching/cool-down

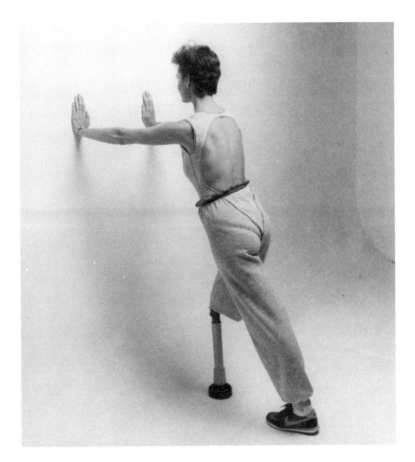

1. Place palms on wall with arms parallel to floor.
2. Bend right knee and place slightly forward. Keep left leg straight.
3. Bend elbows and slowly lean body toward wall. Press forward until you feel the stretch in your left calf. Hold for five to ten seconds. Return to starting position and repeat as able.
4. Alternate sides and repeat as able.

Note: Long periods of inactivity can lead to tightness in the calf and an inability to lift your toes. If your exercise program includes walking again, you can use this exercise to keep the calf stretched and maintained. Remember—as in all stretching exercises—do not bounce.

DESSERT EXERCISE

(Use this at the end of your workout, 'cause you deserve a treat!)

RX1   Take a Trip

Position: get comfortable. Stretch out, close your eyes, or just hug a puppy.

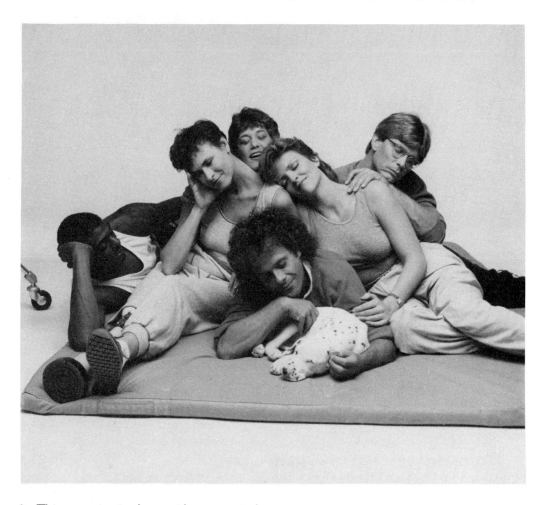

1. This exercise is done with your mind.
2. Take a trip to anyplace in the world—sandy beaches, sunny alps, or even the middle of a clear, blue lake.
3. Close your eyes and listen for the sounds. Feel the gentle breeze as you imagine your body floating above the ground.
4. You've worked hard and you deserve a holiday. Think about how much stronger, firmer, and healthier your body is becoming. Think about how you're gonna be even better tomorrow.

CHAPTER 4
FOOD 4 LIFE

FOOD, GLORIOUS FOOD

"M&Ms are so tiny—how could they hurt? Besides, candy picks me up."

"I can eat all the fruit I want 'cause it keeps my complexion clear."

"Feed a cold and starve a fever."

There are hundreds of silly sayings that pass themselves off as advice on nutrition. And we've all used them! The word "nutrition" has been shoved down our throats for the last decade, and most people still don't know what it is.

Nutrition is the food you swallow and how that body of yours uses it. If you have a piece of melon in the morning, it can be a religious experience; but a doughnut can turn into fat that'll hang out of your Calvin Kleins like folds of drapery fabric.

Maybe you think that because you have a medical or physical challenge you have "special permission" to ignore nutrition and reward yourself with anything your little heart desires. WRONG! I hate to be the one to break it to you, but in this category you're just like everybody else. So join the club. In most cases, your body (especially your heart) responds to food exactly like every other body. "Food in" has to equal "energy out"—or you get covered with fat. Besides, I don't have to remind you that *your* carrying excess weight is the *worst!* Every time you lift a leg, every time you lift an arm, every time you get in and out of your bathtub, you're carrying more dead weight, to put it bluntly, than anybody else. And you've gotta get rid of it!!

That was the bad news.

Here's the good news: NUTRITION IS NOT A FOUR-LETTER WORD.

If I handed you a nutrition quiz, you'd probably get an "A" on it. If I went with you to a supermarket, you'd probably choose all of the "right foods." You know all of the warnings about sugar and cholesterol, and you know that veggies are good for you. You have this knowledge—you just don't use it. Besides, not much in our society supports the concept of good nutrition. Look at school lunch programs, grocery stores, menus in restaurants, or the mass media. Most of us are taught to eat *one* thing and then asked to buy *another*. You have lousy eating habits because you've *learned* them, but now you can learn and practice a new way of eating.

It's the practice that'll really make the difference. Remember when you could eat only one piece of pizza? And then with a little practice you could manage two or three pieces? Practice not only makes perfect—it also makes poundage. But if you practice the *good* things as well as you've practiced the bad things, you're gonna make those new food habits really stick!

Or maybe you don't know all there is about nutrition and exercise. That doesn't matter, 'cause we're gonna teach you the right way to feed and exercise your body.

You're in a wheelchair, you have braces, you're missing a limb, or you have a lung problem. Whatever—you have to know up front that if you go on a temporary *diet,* you'll lose weight, but you'll probably gain it right back. You've just read Chapter Three and you know how you can move that body of yours. Now you have to learn how to feed it—for the rest of your life. All bodies are different, but having a physical challenge makes you even *more* unique. So while a so-called able-bodied person needs to know about proper nutrition, you need to know *even more!*

Without a strong nutritional education to fall back on, you will continue to make the same stupid food mistakes that every-one always does. And besides, the more you learn about food, the less you'll turn to it during times of emotional stress. Using food to relieve stress is very easy. You're depressed because you see people running, playing golf, whatever, and you can't even walk without assistance. So instead, you eat. What you must understand is that food will not grow you a new pair of legs, or get an arm to work better, or make you lighter in your wheelchair.

You probably have every right to be emotional—you didn't come out like the storybooks said—your *this* or your *that* doesn't work the way it was supposed to. But some people turn emotion into bitterness and carry it around with them for a long time. You could be fifty years old and still bitter about an accident that happened thirty years ago. If this is true for you, it's time to come out of the past and start working right now to make every day you're on this earth just a little bit better.

How To DETERMINE YOUR IDEAL WEIGHT

Insurance companies make money when they can accurately guess how long people will live. And since obesity cuts short anybody's life, statisticians within the insurance industry spend a lot of time figuring out how much people *should* weigh. They fly around the country, weighing, measuring, and reading death notices. After gathering all this data, they estimate what seems to be an "ideal" weight for each age and height. Now, you must realize that none of these numbers are set in stone. Moses did not endorse this stuff. And because ther're so many variables when you have a physical challenge, nobody has yet come up with a chart just for you. The following height and weight chart was prepared for the able-bodied population, but even so, it's a good starting point. Chances are you will need to weigh slightly less than what the chart indicates.

1983 Metropolitan Height & Weight Tables

Weights at ages 25-59 based on lowest mortality. Weight in pounds according to frame (in indoor clothing weighing 5 lbs. for men and 3 lbs. for women; shoes with 1" heels).

Metropolitan Insurance Companies

Metropolitan Life Insurance Company
Health and Safety Education Division

1983 METROPOLITAN HEIGHT AND WEIGHT TABLES

	MEN					WOMEN			
Height Feet Inches		Small Frame	Medium Frame	Large Frame		Height Feet Inches	Small Frame	Medium Frame	Large Frame
5	2	128-134	131-141	138-150	4	10	102-111	109-121	118-131
5	3	130-136	133-143	140-153	4	11	103-113	111-123	120-134
5	4	132-138	135-145	142-156	5	0	104-115	113-126	122-137
5	5	134-140	137-148	144-160	5	1	106-118	115-129	125-140
5	6	136-142	139-151	146-164	5	2	108-121	118-132	128-143
5	7	138-145	142-154	149-168	5	3	111-124	121-135	131-147
5	8	140-148	145-157	152-172	5	4	114-127	124-138	134-151
5	9	142-151	148-160	155-176	5	5	117-130	127-141	137-155
5	10	144-154	151-163	158-180	5	6	120-133	130-144	140-159
5	11	146-157	154-166	161-184	5	7	123-136	133-147	143-163
6	0	149-160	157-170	164-188	5	8	126-139	136-150	146-167
6	1	152-164	160-174	168-192	5	9	129-142	139-153	149-170
6	2	155-168	164-178	172-197	5	10	132-145	142-156	152-173
6	3	158-172	167-182	176-202	5	11	135-148	145-159	155-176
6	4	162-176	171-187	181-207	6	0	138-151	148-162	158-179

Copyright 1983 Metropolitan Life Insurance Company   Source of basic data: 1979 Build Study, Society of Actuaries and Association of Life Insurance Medical Directors of America, 1980.

Courtesy of Statistical Bulletin, Metropolitan Life Insurance Company

Once you have a pretty good idea of your ideal weight, there's a neat little formula for determining how many calories you may eat as you safely work toward and then maintain that weight. A lot of weight loss organizations and food plans only count calories. But that's not enough, 'cause your body is more complicated than that. If you want to look and feel better, live longer, and have more energy—you must coordinate calories WITH activity. And so you're gonna learn how many calories are right—not for Raquel Welch or Arnold Schwarzenegger—but for you and your lifestyle.

First, you need to determine how many "basal" calories your body needs. These are the calories necessary for basic maintenance of your heart, lungs, digestive system, etc. To find this number, multiply your ideal body weight by ten. As an example, let's say that you're a woman, five feet four inches tall, and with a small frame. The chart says that an able-bodied person of that height and bone size should weigh 114-127 pounds. Let's go for the average and estimate your ideal weight at about 121.

$$121 \text{ (ideal weight)} \times 10$$
$$= 1,210 \text{ (basal calories)}$$

Next, you must determine how many calories you burn in activity. The more active you are, the more calories your body needs. You find this number by multiplying your ideal weight by something called an activity index. Check the list below and see what value you should give your activity level:

1. bedrest
2. very limited activity
3. no physical exercise (sedentary)
4. moderate exercise (whenever it occurs to you)
5. aerobic exercise, three times per week
6. aerobic exercise, four times per week
7. aerobic exercise, five times per week
8. aerobic exercise, six times per week
9. aerobic exercise, seven times per week
10. major movement (for example, a marathoner)

Continuing our example, let's say that you exercise three times each week. So give yourself a "5."

121 (ideal weight) × 5 (activity index) = 605 (activity calories)

We're almost there—just one more calculation. Now, to determine how many calories you should eat each day, add basal calories to activity calories.

1,210 (basal calories) + 605 (activity calories) = 1,815 (daily caloric intake)

Now, the first thing you're gonna do after figuring this out is faint. You've been taught for the last thousand years that you must eat a very small number of calories to lose weight. And I know that I used to believe the same thing. I've taken shots made from the urine of a pregnant cow and eaten 500 calories a day in an attempt to lose weight. But an orangutan can *lose* weight on 500 calories—it just won't *stay* lost!

More important, ALL doctors now agree that crash diets like this are unsafe. NO ONE should eat less than 1,000 calories per day without close medical supervision. That's because it's almost impossible to get a healthy, balanced food program with so few calories. If your numbers work out to 1,000 or less, you can still use this book, but talk with your doctor or registered dietitian for some specific recommendations.

Let's return to our example. Your ideal weight is 121 and you exercise three times a week. You'll probably look at 1,815 calories and say, "Richard, I'll never lose weight eating that many calories!" But you will. And ther're two reasons for this. First, most people have no idea how many calories they really eat. If you honestly counted every snack and nibble, you may find that you're consuming 3,000 or even 4,000 calories a day. Second, different kinds of food react differently within your body. I'm not gonna talk to you about 1,815 calories of jelly-filled doughnuts; I'm gonna teach you what kinds of calories work most efficiently in your body, give you more long-term energy, and make you feel like being more active.

SO WHAT'S THE BEST WAY TO REACH YOUR IDEAL WEIGHT?

Twelve years ago, when I began working with nutrition and exercise, not much was known. There were very few nutritionists out there, and in general, people were not as fussy and concerned about the food they fed themselves. Nutrition wasn't always taught in school, and it was hard to get this knowledge. Usually, you had to get elected, go to Washington as a congressman, and get a committee briefing from the Food and Drug Administration. But I was lucky enough—*not* to run for office, mind you—to be at the right lecture at the right time, meet the right doctors, and learn about the kinds of food your body needs.

The most important thing I learned is that what you may have thought about nutrition ten or twelve years ago isn't necessarily true. There's a certain amount of basic information—like candy has sugar in it and it could put you in a coma, or an apple is okay because it comes off a tree and God made it. But otherwise, our attitudes about nutrition have matured. We know, for example, how someone should eat if he exercises and which foods contain "nutritionally worthless" calories.

Using experience and this new information, I created the FOOD 4 LIFE program. This isn't just a diet where you eat your plate of lettuce and settle in to watch *Laverne & Shirley* reruns. The FOOD 4 LIFE program includes a scientific formulation of how much and what kind of foods you should eat in relationship to the kind and amount of exercise you do. In this way, you can be sure that you're getting the amount of calories, protein, carbohydrates, fats, etc. that are right for you.

The FOOD 4 LIFE program is a way of looking at food for the rest of your life. The number 4 represents those four things we all need to monitor the most: cholesterol, sugar, salt, and fat.

Most people think CHOLESTEROL is a fatty substance that can line the insides of your arteries as mold can grow in a garden hose. But actually, cholesterol more closely resembles an alcohol. It's an essential part of all cells of your body, especially those that make up your brain, spinal cord, and nerves. It's a major ingredient of bile (the stuff that helps digest food), and it helps manufacture your body's supply of natural cortisone and sex hormones. The cholesterol in the deep layers of your skin keeps you from being poisoned when you touch lots of toxic substances, and it helps regulate perspiration on hot August days. But too much cholesterol can be deadly. The reasons for this are still unclear, but even though scientists don't exactly know how or why, cholesterol does seem to attract fatty substances that *can* accumulate in our blood vessels and cause lots of problems. Until they figure it all out, the best bet is to cut down the amount of cholesterol you consume. Some foods high in cholesterol are egg yolks, animal fats (like those found in red meats, gravies, and lard), and dairy products (like cheese, butter, and whole milk).

There's absolutely no doubt that SUGAR makes you crazy. It artificially stimulates your brain and then causes you to "crash" just like somebody who buys an illegal drug from some guy on a street corner. And the refined sugars you find in processed foods are the worst!

SALT is so necessary for life that in some parts of the world it's still used as money. But too much salt can contribute to high blood pressure, kidney disease, and strokes. Come on, 'fess up, what foods do you oversalt? Corn on the cob? Lima beans? Do you salt your watermelon? I mean, who would ever think that cute little girl with the umbrella on the blue box was gonna cause so many problems?

And because so much of it is hidden in canned foods, frozen foods, and any prepared food, most of us eat a lot of *hidden* salt. For example, when you go to a restaurant, most of the salad dressings, gravies, and sauces have already been "presalted." So even before you pull out your napkin, you have too much salt on your food.

You know all of this but you still grab the saltshaker as you're sitting down in your chair, right? And why do you do that? I know. You're gonna try to tell me that salt *intensifies* the taste of your food. But this is a "learned" taste. Slowly decrease the salt you use and soon you'll wonder how you ever dumped that stuff on your plate.

FATS are necessary to lubricate our bodies, but remember that these fats are just like the fat you're trying to get rid of. They're found in things like butter, margarine, salad dressings, AND ALL FRIED FOODS.

These are the basic "killers," but don't despair. Ther're lots of delicious ways you can feed your body and still keep to the FOOD 4 LIFE program. Enjoy life. Get excited! Just don't celebrate with a chocolate layer cake.

Repeat after me: "The FOOD 4 LIFE program is not for two weeks (snitching on Sundays allowed)—the FOOD 4 LIFE program is for the *rest* of my life."

It's true. Once you learn about the foods you can eat with no guilt—and once your body starts telling you how much better it feels about your new habits—you'll probably never want to eat junk food again. (Well, maybe once in a while, like when your bowling league has its annual barbecue.)

If you wanna lose weight, you have to put up your food antennae. You have to look at all kinds of "danger zones." If, for example, you're watching television and you pick up a bowl of peanuts, ther're about 1,500 calories in that bowl. That's more calories than some people need for an entire day!

MY OH MY, I LOVE IT FRIED
—an essay by R.S.

Anything tastes good fried. You can take the ugliest vegetable in your refrigerator, and once you cover it with batter and deep-fry that sucker, it takes on a whole new life. I could fry cement and eat it. I love batter. But when you think batter, think buns. And don't tell me that after you fry something you blot away the fat with a paper towel. Blotting fried food is about as effective as putting blush on a Barbie doll. Start poaching and broiling food instead of frying it! If you have to add butter or grease to something to make it taste good, you know you're in trouble!

All of the food you have ever tasted in your entire life can be organized into three categories: protein, carbohydrates, and fats. A good rule of thumb is that each day you should eat:

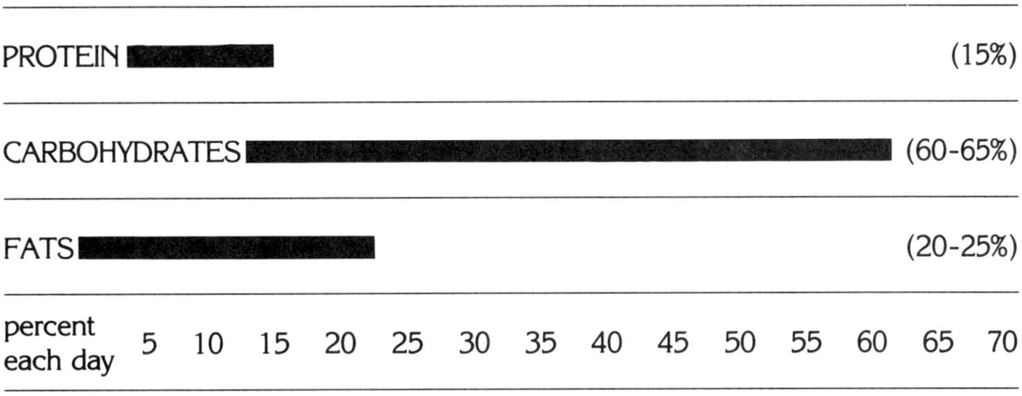
PROTEIN
(15%)
CARBOHYDRATES
(60-65%)
FATS
(20-25%)
percent each day
5 10 15 20 25 30 35 40 45 50 55 60 65 70

PROTEINS have been called the building blocks of our bodies. You get protein from meat, dairy products, fish, poultry, beans, rice, and vegetables. But most protein foods are very high in calories, cholesterol, and fat. A lot of us eat much more protein than our bodies can handle. One adult's serving of protein should be just three and a half *ounces!* I'll bet that surprised you. That's because we're used to seeing much bigger food portions. You got to a restaurant and order the broiled orange roughy, 'cause you know that fish is good for you. When the waiter proudly brings your plate, it's full of ten or twelve ounces of fish! That's enough for the Seventh Fleet.

The same is true with meat or chicken. Yes, this is protein, and, yes, it is good for you. But if you are eating more than three and a half ounces, you're also getting too much protein and fat. The FOOD 4 LIFE food plan will teach you how much is *too much* of a good thing.

And by the way, leading health organizations suggest that you eat red meat only once or twice a week, concentrating instead on the proteins in fish, poultry, and grains.

CARBOHYDRATES (sugars and starches) are either *unrefined* (found in fruits, vegetables, and grains) or *refined* (found in processed foods).

When we leave carbohydrates in an unrefined state, they're pretty good for us. This means leaving the peel on fruits and vegetables and keeping the rice brown, just like God made them for us.

Refined carbohydrates, on the other hand, seem to be our dietary downfall. These are the foods we have created to be *accessories* to natural food. Long, long ago somebody felt the need to make food look "pretty." Enter the accessories, like cakes, pies, candy, ice cream, pretzels, potato chips, cookies, white bread, and pastry. It wasn't enough to have a piece of protein on your plate, a vegetable, a grain dish, and a piece of fruit. Suddenly, natural food looked naked without its accessories. Serve a solitary sandwich to somebody and you'll hear, "Got any chips?"

FATS. Remember our little graph?

Twenty to 25 percent of your daily diet should be fats. I've already warned you about fats, but did you know that 40 to 45 percent of the average American's daily diet is made up of fats! You can tell you're in trouble when the food slides down your throat. That's what the butter and the oil do. They coat the food with a roller-coaster glaze so it can glide down your throat. When people eat fast foods and processed foods, they're just sliding food down their throats for breakfast, lunch and dinner. When you look at the diets of other countries you see that they contain only 10 percent fat! And here we are sliding 40 or 45 percent down our gullets each day! We should be ashamed.

Fat is also present in many "natural" foods. Avocados are loaded with fat. (I know they're your favorite. I know you could just smear guacamole all over your body, but I'm telling you the truth here!) And those sweet little olives that grow on trees like fruit—you know, the ones you suck the pimiento out of— those things can be real body busters. Nuts of all kinds are very high in fat content. Just go to a grocery and look at one of those natural brands of peanut butter. Without special chemicals to keep it from separating, all of the fat rises to the top of the jar. Finally, please don't forget chicken skin (especially when it's crispy lickin' good) or creamy white swirls in the most expensive meats. If you eat fat, your body makes fat. And my friends, the fat on your body is just like that thick yellow chicken fat that makes you gag.

IT'S NOT ONLY WHAT—IT'S ALSO HOW MUCH

The FOOD 4 LIFE program is based on LIFE SERVINGS. *How much* you eat is just as important as *what* you eat. You can gain weight by eating even good foods to excess. A sliver leads to a slab; a slab leads to a slob. The first thing you've got to do is admit that you eat too much food and that many of the foods you eat are full of empty, worthless calories. Until you learn how to eat just the right amount of food to give you the energy you need, you'll always be overweight. A lot of people go on fad diets and lose a lot of weight quickly, but once they return to enormous food servings they gain the weight right back.

But how much is a reasonable portion? How much is too much? Maybe you *really* don't know. You go to a restaurant, for example, and you eat just what somebody puts in front of you. Or you judge food servings by the size of the plates in your cupboard—you just pile on food until the plate's full! Now you must learn a whole different way of looking at the *amount* of food you're eating.

The following FOOD 4 LIFE exchange chart lists examples of each food group and the LIFE SERVINGS you should eat. Pay particular attention to the measurements, 'cause you're gonna be surprised. You know, ther're some things we like to measure; things like vanilla extract or pink laxatives are very carefully dripped into the teaspoon. We take that spoon and measure every last drop of cough syrup, but when it comes to maple syrup we just guess at what a tablespoon *ought* to be.

And notice, for example, that if you adore cheddar cheese you can still eat it—you just need to limit your portion to one and a half ounces per LIFE SERVING. Or if you've been mounding your spaghetti to rival Mt. Vesuvius, please note that three-quarters to one cup is one LIFE SERVING.

The foods on our list are divided into basic food groups, and each LIFE SERVING within a specific group can be interchanged with other foods in the same group. For example, one LIFE SERVING of bread may be: half a bagel, one slice of bread, half a muffin, *or* four pieces of Melba Toast.

Food 4 Life Exchange Chart

Milk/Dairy Products
(1 Life Serving= 85-110 calories)

1 cup	Buttermilk	
1 cup	1% Lowfat Milk	
1 cup	Skim Milk	
1 oz.	Swiss Cheese	
1-1/2 oz.	Mozzarella Cheese, part skim	
1/4 cup	Parmesan or Romano Cheese, grated	
1/3 cup	Ricotta Cheese, part skim	

	Additional Choices	Life Serving Equivalents
1 cup	Whole Milk	1 Milk and 1 "A" Bonus
1 cup	2% Lowfat Milk	1 Milk and 1/2 "A" Bonus
1 cup	Lowfat Chocolate Milk	1 Milk and 1 "A" Bonus
1 cup	Hot Cocoa, whole milk	1 Milk and 2 "A" Bonus
1 cup	Lowfat or Whole Yogurt, plain	1 Milk and 1/2 "A" Bonus
1 cup	Lowfat Yogurt, flavored	1 Milk and 1-1/2 "A" Bonus
1 cup	Lowfat Yogurt, fruited	1 Milk and 2 "A" Bonus
1-1/2 oz.	Bleu Cheese	1 Milk and 1 "A" Bonus
2-1/2 oz.	Camembert Cheese	1 Milk and 2 "A" Bonus
1-1/2 oz.	Cheddar Cheese	1 Milk and 1 "A" Bonus
2 oz.	Cheese Spread	1 Milk and 1 "A" Bonus
1 cup	Cottage Cheese, 1% fat	1 Milk and 1 "A" Bonus
1 cup	Cottage Cheese, creamed	1 Milk and 2 "A" Bonus
2 oz.	Feta Cheese	1 Milk and 1 "A" Bonus
1-1/2 oz.	Gouda Cheese	1 Milk and 1 "A" Bonus
1-1/4 oz.	Monterey Jack Cheese	1 Milk and 1/2 "A" Bonus
2 oz.	Mozzarella cheese, whole milk	1 Milk and 1 "A" Bonus
1-1/4 oz.	Muenster Cheese	1 Milk and 1/2 "A" Bonus
1-1/2 oz.	Port du Salut Cheese	1 Milk and 1 "A" Bonus
1-1/2 oz.	Processed American Cheese	1 Milk and 1 "A" Bonus
1-1/4 oz.	Provolone Cheese	1 Milk and 1/2 "A" Bonus
3/4 cup	Ice Cream or Sherbet	1/2 Milk and 2-1/2 "A" Bonus
1 cup	Ice Milk	1/2 Milk and 2 "A" Bonus

Fats and "A" Bonus* Foods
(1 Life Serving= 40-90 calories)

2 tsp.	Butter, Margarine
2 tsp.	Vegetable Oil
2 tsp.	Mayonnaise
2 tsp.	Salad Dressing, regular
2 tbsp.	Coffee Whitener, liquid
2 tbsp.	Coffee Whitener, powdered
1 tbsp.	Cream, light or heavy
2 tbsp.	Brie Cheese
1 tbsp.	Cream Cheese
2 tbsp.	Half & Half
2 tbsp.	Sour Cream
2 tbsp.	Whipped Cream, unsweetened
3 tbsp.	Whipped Topping, dairy or nondairy
2 tbsp.	Sauce, cheese, cream
2 tbsp.	Gravy
3 tbsp.	Sweet & Sour Sauce
1/3 cup	Barbecue Sauce
2 tbsp.	Seasoned Coating Mix
2 small	Sweet Gherkin Pickles
2 tbsp.	Coconut, shredded
10	Olives
10	Almonds
4 large	Cashews
10 large	Peanuts
2 large	Pecans, whole
2 medium	Walnuts, whole
1 tbsp.	Sunflower Seeds
1 medium	Cookie
1/2 cup	Fruit-flavored Gelatin
1 small	Sugar-type Cone for Ice Cream
6 large	Jelly Beans
4 tsp.	Jelly, Jam
4 tsp.	Sugar, white or brown
1 tbsp.	Honey or Syrup
1 tbsp.	Dessert Topping, butterscotch, hot fudge, lemon, etc.
6 fl. oz.	Breakfast or Soft Drinks, noncarbonated
6 fl. oz.	International Flavored Coffee
8 fl. oz.	Beer, light
1/2 fl. oz.	Brandies, Cordials
1 fl. oz.	Gin, Rum, Vodka, Whiskey
3 fl. oz.	Wine or Sherry, dry
4 fl. oz.	Wine, light

*"A" Bonus foods are foods you can use as rewards for a grade A job of staying on your food plan.

Or Substitute

1 portion	Breads/Cereals/Starchy Foods
2 portions	Fruits
1/2 portion	Milk/Dairy Products
3 portions	Vegetables
1/2 portion	Meat/Poultry/Fish

Meat/Poultry/Fish
(1 Life Serving= 110–150 calories)

Cooked with visible fat removed-broiled, roasted, or baked

2 oz.	Beef, very lean chuck or ground beef, corned beef, flank steak, rib eye, round, rump, sirloin
2 oz.	Chicken/Turkey, Dark meat, no skin
3 oz.	Chicken/Turkey, white meat, no skin
4 oz.	Crab, Lobster
2 oz.	Fish–fatty, herring, mackerel
3 oz.	Fish–medium fat, bluefish, salmon, swordfish
4 oz.	Fish–lowfat, cod, flounder, haddock, halibut, sole
2 oz.	Ham, Canadian Bacon, Chopped Ham, Ham & Cheese Loaf
4 oz.	95% Fat-Free Ham
2 oz.	Lamb, leg, loin roast or chops, shoulder
2 oz.	Liver, Heart, Kidney, Sweetbreads
2 oz.	Meatloaf, Meatballs
2 oz.	Pork, loin, picnic, Boston butt
2 oz.	Veal, cutlets, leg, loin, rib, shank
3 oz.	90% Fat-Free Luncheon Meat
3 slices	Chicken or Turkey Roll
10 medium	Clams, Scallops, Oysters, Mussels
2	Eggs
2 slices	Salami, beef, pork, turkey
5 medium	Sardines, canned, drained
10 large	Shrimp
1 piece	Tofu (soybean curd) (2-1/2" × 2-1/2" × 2")
1/2 cup	Tuna, canned, drained

	Additional Choices	Life Serving Equivalents
4 strips	Bacon	1/2 Meat and 2 "A" Bonus
2 slices	Bologna	1 Meat and 1 "A" Bonus
1 link	Bratwurst	1 Meat and 2 "A" Bonus
3 slices	Braunschweiger	1 Meat and 1 "A" Bonus
4 links	Breakfast Sausage	1 Meat and 1-1/2 "A" Bonus
2 oz.	Deviled Ham	1 Meat and 1 "A" Bonus
1 medium	Frank or Wiener	1 Meat and 1 "A" Bonus
2 oz.	Ground Beef, regular	1 Meat and 1/2 "A" Bonus
6 slices	Hard Salami	1 Meat and 2 "A" Bonus
1 link	Italian Sausage	1 Meat and 1-1/2 "A" Bonus
1 link	Knockwurst	1 Meat and 1-1/2 "A" Bonus
2 slices	Luncheon Meat	1 Meat and 1/2 "A" Bonus
2 patties	Pork Sausage	1 Meat and 1-1/2 "A" Bonus
2 oz.	Spare Ribs, lean	1 Meat and 1-1/2 "A" Bonus

Freebies
(1 Life Serving= less than 15 calories)

Coffee, black		**Limit to two**	
Tea, plain		**portions**	
Bouillon		**per day:**	
Diet/Sugar-free Soft	1	Dill Pickle	
Drinks	4 slices	Bread 'n' Butter	
Club Soda		Pickles	
Water	1 tbsp.	Catsup,	
Artificial Sweetener		Cocktail Sauce	
Mustard	1 tbsp.	Horseradish	
Lemon or Lime Juice	1 tbsp.	Low-calorie	
Pimiento		Salad Dressing	
Soy Sauce, Vinegar	2 tsp.	Relish, sweet	
Vinegar	1/2 cup	Low-calorie Gelatin	
Salt & Pepper	2 tsp.	Reduced-calorie	
Herbs, basil, bay leaf,		Whipped Topping	
dill, oregano,	1/4 cup	Taco Sauce	

parsley, etc.
Spices, chili, cloves, cinnamon, curry, sage, etc.

1 small	Wafer-type Cone for Ice Cream

Vegetables
(1 Life Serving= 15–30 calories)

1/2 cup raw or cooked	Artichoke Hearts		Wax Beans
	Asparagus	1/3 cup	Tomato Sauce
	Bean Sprouts	1 cup raw	Beet Greens
	Beets	or	Cabbage
	Broccoli	cooked	Cauliflower
	Brussels Sprouts		Celery
	Carrots		Cucumber
	Collard Greens		Green Pepper
	Eggplant		Mushrooms
	Green Beans		Radishes
	Kale		Summer Squash
	Mustard Greens		Zucchini Squash
	Onions	2 cups raw	Endive
	Sauerkraut		Lettuce
	Spinach, cooked		Spinach
	Tomato Juice		Watercress
	Tomatoes		**See Breads/**
	Turnip		**Cereals/Starchy**
	Turnip Greens		**Foods list for**
	Vegetable Juice Cocktail		**"starchy" vegetables**

Breads/Cereals/Starchy Foods
(1 Life Serving= 60–80 calories)

1/2	Bagel, Matzoh	1/2 cup cooked	Oatmeal, Grits, Farina, Cream of Rice, Whole Wheat Cereal
1 small	Biscuit		
1 slice	Bread		
2 medium	Bread Sticks, plain		
1/4 cup	Breadcrumbs, dry	1/2 cup	Ready-to-Eat Cereals, except granola-types
2 squares	Graham Crackers		
1/2	Roll, hard, hamburger, hot dog	1/4 cup	Beans, baked, garbanzo
1 small	Roll, dinner, crescent	1/2 cup cooked	Pasta, macaroni, spaghetti, noodles
1/2	Muffin, blueberry, bran, corn, English, plain	1/2 medium	Potato, baked, boiled
1/2 large	Pita Bread	1/2 cup	Potato, mashed
3 cups popped	Popcorn	1/3 cup cooked	Rice
10	Pretzel Rings, single	1/4 cup	Sweet Potato, or Yam
6	Saltines or other small crackers	1/3 cup	Corn, Black-eyed Peas, Lentils, Lima Beans
4 pieces	Melba Toast		
1	Tortilla, 6 inch	1/2 cup	Peas, Peas & Carrots, Winter Squash
2	Zwieback		
		1/2 large ear	Corn on the Cob

Fruits
(1 Life Serving= 30–50 calories)

	Fresh, canned, or frozen unsweetened fruits	1/2 small	Grapefruit
		1/2 cup	Grapefruit Juice
		12	Grapes
1 small	Apple	1/10	Honeydew Melon
1/2 medium	Apple	1 small	Nectarine
1/3 cup	Apple Juice	1/2 cup	Mandarin Oranges
1/2 cup	Applesauce	1 small	Orange
1/2 cup	Apricot Halves	1/3 cup	Orange Juice
1/3 cup	Apricot Nectar	1 medium	Peach
2 medium	Apricots	1/2 cup	Peach Halves or Slices

1/8	Avocado	1/2 medium	Pear		
1/2 small	Banana				
1/2 cup	Blueberries	1/2 cup	Pear Halves or Slices		
1/4	Cantaloupe	1/2 cup	Pineapple Chunks		
10	Cherries	1/3 cup	Pineapple Juice		
1/2 cup	Citrus Sections	2 small	Plums		
1/3 cup	Cranberry Juice	1/4 cup	Prune Juice		
2	Dates, Prunes	2 tbsp.	Raisins		
1	Fig, dried or fresh	3/4 cup	Strawberries		
1/2 cup	Fruit Cocktail	1 medium	Tangerine		
1/3 cup	Grape Juice	1 cup	Watermelon		

Combination Foods

		Life Serving Equivalents			
3 slices	French Toast	3 Bread, 1/2 Meat, and 1 "A" Bonus	1/6 pie	Quiche, plain	1 Bread, 1/2 Meat, 1 Milk, and 1 "A" Bonus
4 medium	Pancakes	2 Bread, 1/2 Meat, and 1/2 "A" Bonus	2	Tacos, beef or chicken	2 Bread, 1-1/2 Meat, 1 Veg., 1/2 Milk, and 1/2 "A" Bonus
3 small	Waffles	2 Bread, 1/2 Meat, and 1 "A" Bonus	1/2 cup	Bread Stuffing	1-1/2 Bread and 1 "A" Bonus
1	Burrito, beef & bean	2 Bread, 1/2 Meat, and 1 "A" Bonus	10 medium	French Fries	1 Bread and 1-1/2 "A" Bonus
1 cup	Chicken Chow Mein	1 Meat and 2 Veg.	1/2 cup	Seasoned Rice Mix	1-1/2 Bread and 1/2 "A" Bonus
1 cup	Chili with Beans	2 Bread, 1 Meat, 1 Veg., and 1/2 "A" Bonus	1/2 cup	Coleslaw	1/2 Veg. and 1 "A" Bonus
3"×3"×3"	Lasagna	1 Bread, 1 Meat, 2 Veg., 2 Milk, and 1 "A" Bonus	1/2 cup	Macaroni or Potato Salad	1 Bread and 1 "A" Bonus
1 cup	Macaroni and Cheese	2 Bread, 2 Milk, and 1 "A" Bonus	1/2 cup	Custard, baked	1/2 Meat, 1/2 Milk and 1/2 "A" Bonus
1/6 large pie	Pizza, cheese	1 Bread, 1 Veg., 1/2 Milk, and 1 "A" Bonus	1/2 cup	Fruit, canned, sweetened	1 Fruit and 1 "A" Bonus
			1/2 cup	Pudding, regular	1/2 Milk and 2 "A" Bonus
			1/2 cup	Pudding, reduced-calorie	1/2 Milk and 1/2 "A" Bonus

Soups, prepared with water

8 fl. oz.	Chicken Noodle	1/2 Bread and 1/2 "A" Bonus
7-1/2 fl. oz.	Chunky Beef	1 Bread, 1/2 Meat, and 1 Veg.
8 fl. oz.	Clam Chowder, Manhattan	1 Bread
8 fl. oz.	Cream of Mushroom	1/2 Bread and 1-1/2 "A" Bonus
8 fl. oz.	Split Pea with Ham	1 Bread, 1/2 Meat, and 1/2 "A" Bonus
8 fl. oz.	Tomato	1 Bread and 1/2 Veg.
8 fl. oz.	Vegetable	1 Bread and 1/2 Veg.

Time for a little review. How much is a reasonable LIFE SERVING?

—An entire pizza is too much.

—A reasonable portion of bread is one slice or one small dinner roll. We're not talking the entire loaf of Italian here.

—If you decide to eat a ground-beef patty (remember, keep the servings of red meat down to one or two per week), you probably would hold the bun without being told. But a patty that's six inches in diameter is too big. Something that size doesn't even qualify for a cute little name like "patty." Three inches in diameter and a half inch thick is plenty. If your protein is coming to your plate by weight, three and a half ounces is a reasonable amount.

—An entire chicken is too much. The only bird that qualifies for the whole-bird portion is a baby quail or a Cornish hen. (And even then we're talking "guts-empty," broiled, not stuffed with buttered breadcrumbs.) One chicken breast or one leg and a thigh would be considered a reasonable amount.

—There's been a lot of controversy about how many eggs you should eat. Eggs can be a very good source of protein, but just to be on the safe side, limit eggs to one or two a week.

Personally, I don't eat eggs very often. You know what the yolk is, right? An egg yolk is that cute little yellow part that has all the flavor. God made egg yolks and then said, "How could I ever top this?" That precious little egg yolk contains 250 milligrams of cholesterol! So think about your heart and arteries the next time you think about eggs. Besides, who can just stop with the egg? Eggs lead to hash browns; hash browns lead to buttered toast; and you know what buttered toast leads to.

—Unless we're talking grapes or berries, only one piece of fruit is reasonable. Six apples, a crate of oranges—you can get too much of a good thing with lots of fruit. In the case of grapes or berries, three-quarters of a cup, please.

—If you fix yourself a bowl of cereal and it's filled so full that it looks like the Leaning Tower of Pisa with the bananas falling to the side, you are eating enough cereal for the Waltons.

—Having fish? Remember, you only need 3½ ounces after cooking (that's about ¾ of a cup).

—When you pick up a potato at the supermarket, get one that's small and firm. Save the Idaho County Fair winners for somebody else.

—Butter? You're allowed a certain number of fat servings each day. Your body needs a little bit of fat, but not the amounts you're probably giving it now. One LIFE SERVING of butter is one teaspoon. But while most of us can have three LIFE SERVINGS of fat per day, some people put more butter on a single morning's toast than their bodies need for an entire week! Mayonnaise is the same thing as butter when it comes to planning your FOOD 4 LIFE program. And you know darn well that when you're fluffin' up that tuna salad you add more than three teaspoons of mayo!! In fact, you're probably using *ten* teaspoons. And those extra seven teaspoons of mayo are turning into your extra pounds!

—God bless veggies. But unfortunately, you still have to watch LIFE SERVINGS. Too many vegetables can also put on weight. Some vegetables have relatively few calories and thus have relatively larger LIFE SERVINGS. You saw them in the food charts, but some of the more popular are lettuce, celery, cabbage, brussels sprouts (Have you ever wondered if they're just little baby cabbages passing themselves off as brussels sprouts?), broccoli, onions, green peppers, squash (green or yellow), beets, and spinach.

There are some vegetables you have to be careful about: mainly the ol' beans and peas, corn, white potatoes, sweet potatoes, and carrots. About a half to three-quarters of a cup would be a reasonable portion.

—Finally, look out for the Foolers. These are the tiny little guys in cute little packages that pack away big, big calorie counts. As in: "I don't know why I can't lose weight, I only sneaked one or two. . . ." The Foolers are bubble gum, breath mints, those packets of Knott's Berry Farm jelly that some nice person put on your restaurant table, the candy that grows on hotel pillows, and the peanut butter and jelly crusts the kids leave on their plates. Everybody falls for a Fooler now and then, and you will, too. Just be careful—they can be very seductive.

As you consider the portions of food you should eat, remember this about your stomach: Its normal dimension is about the size of your fist. (That stuff below your belt that you call your belly is really fat and overworked intestines. Your stomach is higher up.) When you eat, your stomach swells (as a vacuum-cleaner bag does) to accommodate the volume you cram into it.

YOUR FOOD 4 LIFE DAILY PLAN

Look to the height and weight chart on page 125, multiply your ideal weight by your activity level (see page 126), and calculate how many calories you need to eat. Remember, this is to *maintain* your ideal body weight. If you want to lose weight, you must decrease your calories or increase your activities. Experts estimate that you must consume 500 *fewer* or burn 500 *more* calories EACH day in order to lose a pound of fat a week.

So how many calories should you eat each day? Check one of the following:

— 1,500 to 1,800 calories per day.
— 1,200 to 1,500 calories per day.
— 1,000 to 1,200 calories per day.

The number of calories you need to consume should be carefully distributed throughout the day. For example, don't eat the entire 1,000 calories at breakfast. We've developed three food plans that organize your meals and tell you how many LIFE SERVINGS you should eat from each major food group.

HOW THE FOOD 4 LIFE PLAN WORKS IF YOU SHOULD EAT 1,000 TO 1,200 CALORIES PER DAY

If you're a member of the 1,000 to 1,200 per day club, don't worry. The time has come for you to finally take off and keep off the weight you want to lose. (And I'm not just talking your everyday "lose," folks, I'm talking "drop-off-the-edge-of-the-planet-never-to-be-heard-from-again-lose!" You've tried before and it's always found its way home again. You've given up, I bet, and you think that nobody really cares if you're fat or not. Well, that's not true. I care and you do, too, or you wouldn't be reading this book right now. So two people are enough. Don't let either of us down.

Look to Plan A below and see how many and what kinds of LIFE SERVINGS you may choose from the exchange chart listed on pages 131 to 133. If you stick with the FOOD 4 LIFE Plan A, exercise every day, and keep up your mental attitude, you'll reach your ideal weight.

PLAN A
1,000–1,200 Calories

	Milk	Meat	Fat	Bread	Fruit	Veg
Breakfast	1	1	1	1	1	0
Lunch	0	1	1	2	2	0
Dinner	1	2	2	1	1	3
Total	2	4	4	4	4	3

If you are on Plan A, a sample break-fast menu consists of a Hurry-Up Fruit Shake (blend ½ cup plain low-fat yogurt, ¼ tsp. lemon juice, ½ cup strawberries, ¼ cup orange juice, and ⅛ tsp. nutmeg), 1 slice of whole wheat toast, and 1 tea-spoon of butter. Now, that's not nearly as bad as a piece of dry toast and a cup of hot water, is it? And yet, you can still lose weight on this much food.

How the FOOD 4 LIFE Plan Works If You Should Eat 1,200 to 1,500 Calories per Day

You've been fooling yourself for a while, right? Lying to that nice lady who fills in the boxes on your driver's license? Think-ing that you'll eat french fries today at lunch and skip dinner? Promising to start your new diet as soon as the ice cream's all gone? This is the time for honest, new, and wonderful beginnings. Step right up there and learn all about FOOD 4 LIFE Plan B.

If you are on Plan B, a sample lunch menu could include 1 piece of quiche (1 bread serving, ½ meat serving, 1 milk serving, 1 fat serving); 2 ounces of shredded crabmeat; 1 small dinner roll, and 1 teaspoon of butter; ½ cup of sliced tomatoes and a fruit salad made of ½ cup blueberries, ½ of a small banana, ½ cup of mandarin oranges, and 10 cherries. That's quite a feast.

PLAN B
1,200–1,500 Calories

	Milk	Meat	Fat	Bread	Fruit	Veg
Breakfast	1	1	1	2	1	0
Lunch	1	1	2	2	2	1
Dinner	1	3	1	2	1	3
Total	3	5	4	6	4	4

How the FOOD 4 LIFE Plan Works If You Should Eat 1,500 to 1,800 Calories per Day

Nobody understands, do they? You tell your friends that you have to lose five pounds and they throw their napkins at you! But your "few" pounds are as difficult to lose as are someone else's "one hundred and few." You've tried all the fad diets and you lose weight some-times—it just seems to reattach itself the moment you turn your back on it. (And somewhere in the middle of your back-side is usually where it shows up, right?) Well, you can do it this time! You just have to learn to eat Plan C.

If you are on Plan C, you will be amazed at what you can have for dinner. A sample menu could include 10 large shrimp and 1 tablespoon of cocktail sauce; 3 ounces of chicken breast (no skin); 1/3 cup cooked rice; a salad made of ½ cup artichoke hearts, 2 cups mixed lettuce, and ½ cup tomatoes; 4 Melba Toast crackers; 2 teaspoons of salad dressing; ½ cup reduced-calorie vanilla pudding (consisting of 1 milk serving and 1 fat serving) topped with 1 dried fig. That sounds like enough for an army, but look at the very low amount of fat you're consuming! And believe it or not, you *still* have 1 meat and 1 bread serving left over! So if you wanted an evening snack, you could have 5 sardines and three cups of plain popcorn!

When you read the food list on pages 131 to 133, you probably noticed that some foods were made up of combinations of LIFE SERVINGS. For example, a

PLAN C
1,500–1,800 Calories

	Milk	Meat	Fat	Bread	Fruit	Veg
Breakfast	1	1	2	3	1	0
Lunch	1	1	2	2	2	1
Dinner	1	3	2	3	1	3
Total	3	5	6	8	4	4

piece of cheese pizza is a combination of 1 bread serving, 1 vegetable serving, ½ milk serving, and 1 fat serving. You should work combination foods into your daily food plan because they add variety and satisfy you much more than those old "bouillon and diced carrots" diets. But remember, they can be danger zones. Let's say you have one LIFE SERVING of fat in your plan for dinner. Go ahead and eat a bran muffin if you want, but realize that it already contains fat. If you spread on an additional tea-spoon of butter, you are not staying on your plan. And those little "slips" can be what keeps you from losing weight.

There are some final hints about making your FOOD 4 LIFE plan work.

—Don't skip meals and don't overload all your calories into one or two huge meals. Your body can burn calories more efficiently (and thus lose easier) if you eat several small meals each day.

—Learn to recognize an ideal LIFE SERVING. Initially you'll need to measure, but it'll be easier when you can "eyeball" it. Nobody wants to walk around with a set of plastic measuring spoons tied to his belt, so learn to estimate food portions. For example, measure out a half cup of dry macaroni, pour it into the palm of your hand, and remember how it looks and feels. The next time, you can estimate a LIFE SERVING and more easily work FOOD 4 LIFE into *your* life.

—Feel free to move LIFE SERVINGS around in your daily food plans. For example, if you're allowed two bread servings for lunch, you can save one for a mid-afternoon snack.

—Remember, this is not just a weight loss plan; it's a plan to provide you with appropriate nutrients and to get your body to function at its best level. So don't omit any of your allotted LIFE SERVINGS. Many of our moods and emotions are influenced by nutrition, and starving yourself can make you feel and act miserable. Eat the right amounts of the right foods and there's no reason to feel hungry and deprived.

With these FOOD 4 LIFE plans, you are in charge. I'm not gonna give you a list of menus that you *must* eat on the "third Wednesday" of the "fifth week." There are so many wonderful foods out there that you can and should discover for yourself. Who says you have to eat the same breakfast, lunch, and dinner as everybody else? So enjoy the varieties of life. Try an unusual fruit you've never tasted before; don't just stick to the "old standards." When it's time to eat breads, look for the ones that are crunchy and have bran. Try some ethnic bread that you've never tried. Be creative. Maybe one morning you'll take your breakfast bread and melt a little bit of cheese on it. On the next day you may decide to have a waffle and puree a banana for a special "banana syrup." It's delicious and still well within your FOOD 4 LIFE program.

A Day in the Life of a Well-Adjusted FOOD 4 LIFE Plan

BREAKFAST

Breakfast is good for two reasons. First, it gets your energy up and gets your body moving. The fructose in oranges and grapefruit, for example, can give your body a little "natural high." The second reason you should eat breakfast is so that your body will be stimulated to go to the bathroom. This is true of all animals. When you see a dog after its morning walk, it comes back happy, ears up, and bouncing along, 'cause everything's great. It's an important thing for the body to do. Now, if you do not go to the bathroom in the morning, chances are that you do not eat breakfast. And chances are that you will be hostile all day! Look around you; you can always tell the people who have not gone to the bathroom yet. If the mailman comes to the door and he's grumpy—he did not go to the bathroom. If your mother comes downstairs and she's not in a good mood—no bathroom. I mean, let's just take a look at Alexis Carrington. That girl hasn't been to the bathroom for three years!

Breakfast is the best spot to have your fiber for the day. Fiber is that undigestible food material that helps us clean out our digestive systems—sort of a Mother Earth Roto-Rooter system. And fiber is found primarily in the brans and whole grains you eat at breakfast. So eat a nice bowl of cereal (hot or cold), or eat a good, earthy, grainy piece of bread. Forget all about white bread. That's had the fiber processed out so it's almost as good for you as the paper it's wrapped in.

When you're preparing breakfast, again, consider the volume. If you decide to have a glass of juice, take a small glass (½ a cup). After all, 6 to 8 oranges must give their lives to produce an iced-tea tumbler full of juice. Would you consider sitting down and eating 6 to 8 oranges? No, so have your ½ *cup* of juice. Put some crushed ice in it, stick it in the freezer, and make it into a Smoothy-Frosty; sip it slowly and enjoy. You'll freeze your teeth and gums, and the last thing you'll wanna do is eat something fattening.

And while we're on the subject of juice, for heaven's sake, stay away from those canned drinks with 10 percent real fruit! I'm embarrassed for some manufacturers when I read on those cans that a drink is 10 percent fruit juice. What happened to the other 90 percent? Did it walk out of the can? Why am I stuck with just 10 percent?? Stay with natural fruit juice.

Once in a while, treat yourself with a couple of whole grain pancakes or a waffle. (But use a nonstick product to avoid frying.) Pancakes and waffles themselves are fine; it's the two cups of syrup and half a cup of butter that'll kill you. So have a waffle now and then; just use one tablespoon of syrup and skip the butter (you won't even miss it).

LUNCH

Lunch is the meal you eat when your energy level has been depleted by the morning's activities. (Unless, of course, you've skipped breakfast—in which case you find yourself eating out of other people's brown bags.) You've been thinking, working, moving, performing at your job, and exercising, and you're ready to be recharged. And so the purpose of lunch is to rejuvenate and energize. It gets energy to your muscles and brain so that you are alert and ready to continue working. This is the perfect time for vegetables, either in a salad or in a bowl of soup. This is not the perfect time for a nine-course dinner because Anna Maria's birthday falls on a "lunch Wednesday." It's always somebody's birthday, your parents' anniversary, or the opening of a new restaurant. Somebody wants to take you to lunch and you eat anything in sight simply because it's a "freebie."

This may be the spot you choose to have your dairy product, a small piece of hard cheese, a small portion of cottage cheese, or a cup of yogurt. (Stay away from those that are loaded with extra sugar and fruit!)

Lunch should be light, 'cause it's actually a snack. It's not necessary for you to sit down to a three-course meal; your body doesn't need that much only halfway through the day. Too much food, and energies will be drained as you try to digest. You'll get lethargic; you'll get sleepy, and all you'll want to do is curl up with a pillow and a good book. That's what happens in Europe. Those people on the Continent eat huge lunches and then they have to close down all the shops, block off the entrances to the museums, and take a nap. (So, please, if you're saving for a trip to Europe, go shopping in the morning—after all those people have had a good breakfast and gone to the bathroom. You'll get much better deals that way. After lunch, all the prices go up 'cause they don't wanna be bothered.)

DINNER

Dinner time is also a time of rejuvenation, not a time for reward! You know—you work hard all day, you come home tired and hungry, and you expect some kind of Roman banquet or something. You *have* used up a lot of your calories and you do need to be recharged, but what are you going to do *after* dinner? Go outside and build a barn? Chop tomorrow's firewood? No, and neither does anybody else. Years ago, when people spent long hours in hard physical labor, big meals were a necessity. Now all of us are more sedentary. And if you have physical challenges that restrict your movements, you need even less food at the end of the day.

Dinner is the perfect time for a small piece of protein (three and a half ounces of chicken, fish, or meat), a vegetable, and maybe a small salad.

If you've saved a fat allowance, now's the time to treat yourself and put a tablespoon of *real* dressing on that salad.

Diet salad dressings have had most of the fat removed, but look at them closely. That stuff that holds the vinegar and spices together is gum. When you shake a bottle of diet salad dressing and nothing moves, it should tell you that the taste won't move you, either. A tablespoon of a good dressing (even one with oil in it) will be much more satisfying—and if you've followed your program all day, that's not cheating. (Here's a neat trick: add 1-3 tablespoons of lemon juice, water, or vinegar to regular dressing. It'll stretch over more salad and taste terrific! Better yet, make your own low-cal dressing with a little oil, a lot of vinegar, and fresh herbs.)

SOME FOODS NEED SPECIAL ATTENTION

SNACKS

Snacking is only extra calories. The average American consumes 60 percent of his or her daily caloric intake in the form of snacks. Most of the time, these snacks are very low in nutrients and contain only sugar, starch, salt, and fat. Even with all the exercises that you can do, snacking will keep your weight constant.

Everybody needs to reach for something in times of depression or insecurity. The best thing to reach for is another human being. Hugging, touching, and squeezing are totally low-cal. When you turn to a refrigerator, you are really looking for someone to hug or to listen. When I was a kid, I guess one of the real reasons I ate was that food didn't talk back to me. If I got a "B" in chemistry and my mother and father were screaming at me to get an "A," the Oreo cookies in the bag stayed calm. When no one wanted to play with me at school, a peanut butter and jelly sandwich was there. Food would first be in front of me, and then as I ate it, I would bring it into myself and it would become a part of me. That always made me feel safe and warm.

Snacking also fulfills another personal need. It makes noise in our mouths. When we snack and hear the crunch, we're not alone anymore. It's the sound that makes us happy. The sound of food being chewed is consoling, and so that's why most snacks are crispy and crunchy, like potato chips and pretzels and cookies. If you took the snap, crackle, and pop away from it, nobody'd eat that stuff. But why deny yourself something so emotionally satisfying? Either chew pencils or find an *appropriate* snack. If, for example, you're allowed three LIFE SERVINGS of bread, keep one for a snack. Toast it, cut it into little squares, and munch away. Another terrific snack idea is that big bowl of crisp, raw vegetables in ice water. Then when you feel blue or you feel alone or you feel insecure, go to the fridge and make a lot of noise with a carrot stick!

COFFEE AND TEA

Fruit gives you a natural high, and the caffeine in coffee, tea, and cola gives you an unnatural or chemical high. Having a cup of coffee in the morning is not a sin, but when you spend the day consuming five or six cups of coffee, you've got too much caffeine surging through your body. Besides, only 10 percent of Americans drink coffee or tea with nothing

else in it. Are you one of those people, or does a cup of coffee also mean a tablespoon of cream and a couple of sugar cubes? So take that single cup of coffee in the morning and enjoy it, fondle it, cuddle with it, take it for walks with you, and make it your pet for the day. Then for the rest of the day rely upon your own internal energies and enthusiasms.

(By the way, if you find yourself missing coffee on a cold winter afternoon, heat a little apple juice and add a cinnamon stick. It's wonderful!)

ALCOHOL AND DIET DRINKS

Unless you have strict instructions from your doctor, you know that one glass of wine probably won't hurt. But how many people stop at just one?

I also suggest that you limit diet drinks to one per day. I know it's just one calorie, and I've seen Michael Jackson and Lionel Richie skip down the street in their size-three leather pants telling you that Pepsi's okay for you. But while five Cokes can be a thousand calories and five diet Cokes are just five calories, you are filling your body with a lot of chemicals. And we still don't know everything about what those chemicals do. Especially if you are on regular medication, it just makes sense to limit the amount of extra chemicals you consume.

MILK

What is an Oreo without a glass of milk? Most of us were raised on milk; it is a part of our mutual heritage. Long before it was low-fat, non-fat, high-fat, quick-fat, goodbye fat—it was just *milk*. But now we're finding out that some of us are allergic to dairy products. You may be allergic to cheese, milk, and ice cream. I am. Dairy products are mucus forming, and this can be particularly harmful if you have a respiratory condition such as asthma or emphysema. So limit dairy products and, as with coffee, think of them as *treats.*

DESSERTS

Every nutritionist in the world will stand by your side, look at a plate of fruit, and tell you that it takes the place of dessert. Well, it doesn't. I don't care how you cut your fruit, or what pretty bowl you put it in, it doesn't taste like a chocolate mousse. You can even sculpt an apple to *look* like a chocolate mousse and it'll still *taste* like an apple.

I don't expect you to have a carrot with a candle in it for your birthday! *One piece of cake on a special day's not gonna kill you.* But on that special day, look at your LIFE SERVINGS and plan how you're gonna cut back on something else so you can afford a piece of your birthday cake.

CANDY

Uck! Can I make myself any more clear? Candy is sugar, chemicals, and fat; it has absolutely no food value whatsoever. Candy is the stuff you should give your worst enemy, not your lover or your child. If somebody gives you candy, bury it in the yard. (Well, maybe you shouldn't, 'cause you'd probably dig it up after the kids go to bed.)

We're all human, and candy is something that we can't always avoid, but if you find that you're getting that *chocolate urge* more than once a week, just tape a Hershey bar to your hips to remind yourself where that candy is really going.

WATER

Do I have to tell you how important water is? I mean, think for a minute: *20,000 Leagues Under the Sea, Moby Dick,* Palm Springs—"you know who" walked on it. Where would we be without water? Some people say, "You're full of hot air," but that's not true. You're really full of water. In fact, it makes up over 90 percent of your body.

You get a certain amount of water in fruits, vegetables, juices, and even colas. But none of these liquids works as well as plain, ol', out-of-the-tap water for flushing out your body or quenching your thirst. Put some ice in a tall glass of water and stick it in the freezer for ten minutes. When you take it out, we're talking Maui in July. I try to get at least five extra glasses of water each day. (Eight or nine, and I'll admit that I start feeling a little like Noah's Ark.)

NOBODY'S MADE OF STONE

Listen, I wanna tell you something. I have lost one hundred and thirty-seven pounds. But there are times when I would sell my mother for a hot loaf of bread and a stick of butter. I LOVE food and I'll always love food. I hope there's room service in heaven! When I first started traveling to promote my television series, my biggest challenge was breakfast in the hotel room. I'd call room service and say, "Hi, Room Service? Ther're two of us; I'll have one boiled egg and the juice, and my friend will have—What's that you want?—my friend will have two orders of waffles and the French toast." Then, when the man would bring up my food, I'd turn on the shower, yell, "I'll get it, I'll get it!" open the door, and smile.

I am a compulsive eater. And maybe some of you out there are compulsive eaters, too. I know it's not gonna be easy for you at first. Here I am, giving you rules and regulations about breakfast, lunch, and dinner, but, meanwhile, food is always gonna be there. Drive down any highway in your town; it'll be lined with places that are whispering your name. Turn on your television set; they've got the hamburger in that commercial so close to your face that you can get a suntan as you watch it broil. You're the one who's gonna have to change! You're the one who's gonna have to take the responsibility into your own Mr. Knife and Mr. Fork hands. And you're the one who's gonna have to look at food and say, "What's more important? A piece of pecan pie, or my life?"

The choice is up to you. And as I see it, you've got two ways to go. You can either stuff yourself at a hearty last meal and wheel yourself off a bridge, or you can actually make a commitment to change your eating habits. The quality of food that you eat will help determine the quality of life that you'll live.

RICHARD'S LIFE SAVERS

There are some behavior modification tips (I call 'em LIFE SAVERS) that can help you get started on your FOOD 4 LIFE program. These may seem simple at first, but they really do work.

Use smaller plates. When you put your three ounces of chicken and a vegetable on one of those giant, fancy dinner plates, it looks like you've prepared dinner for Olive Oyl. Use smaller plates and your smaller food portions will *look* right.

Use smaller utensils. The same psychology is at work here. There's no reason to lean a giant fork against your shoulder. Big forks hold too much spaghetti, and you don't need that. Get yourself some small forks and start eating small amounts.

Never shop for food on an empty stomach. And if you can shop by yourself, *Never take a friend food shopping.* You've heard it before but it bears repeating: When you shop hungry or you shop with a friend, you end up buying a thousand times more than you need.

Keep your place in restaurants. Your place in a restaurant is as the *customer,* not as the doormat. Think of it the same way you think of a department store. If I go to a department store, pay twenty-five dollars for a new shirt, come home, and find that the collar's ripped, I take the shirt back. I look at food the same way. If I go into a restaurant to plop down hard-earned money, I'm not gonna be intimidated by anybody. I tell the waiter or waitress that I want the fancy rolls and butter removed from the table. Then I look at the menu and say, "I'm on a special food program, can you prepare this without butter? I want this without the cream sauce."

And what about when you go to somebody's house for dinner? There's no reason you have to sit there and play Joan of Arc. When you get the invitation, you can say very sweetly, "I'm on the FOOD 4 LIFE program and I can eat this and this. I'm really looking forward to being with you; should I bring my own dinner? Should I bring all the dinners?" Nine times out of ten the host or hostess will be more than happy to accommodate your needs. And what about that one who gives you an argument? Just start crying on the phone and hang up—she'll feel real bad and call you right back!

Get out of the kitchen. Stop making the kitchen the most important room in your house. Have you seen some of these fancy kitchens? I know people who have office desks and telephones, family entertainment centers, and Cub Scout meetings in their kitchens. These same people are in their refrigerators twenty times a day. What are they doing? Checking to see if somebody stole the food? Checking to see if the light bulb's burned out while their backs were turned?

And what about when you watch TV?! I know what you do during the commercials. You (a) go to the bathroom, (b) go to the kitchen to check the refrigerator, or (c) bother somebody in another room. Why do you check the refrigerator? Do you honestly think the Good Food Fairy left you something? (If she ever does, I want you to call me immediately! We can turn your house into a shrine and make a fortune off the souvenir T-shirts.)

We put a meter on the refrigerator of a family with two children, a cat, and a parrot, and during one day, that refrigerator door was opened 1,100 times! I'll give you a hint: The cat and the parrot didn't do it.

Do not use food for decoration. You do not need to put your coconut cake in a crystal cake saver. Come to think of it, what are you doing with a coconut cake, anyway? Put all food in cupboards and drawers. The same goes for food appliances. Betty Crocker days are over; you have no reason to dress the blender in a cute little cover and keep it close at hand. Out of sight, off of thighs!

Purge your pantry. Go immediately to your cupboards, put on a tape of Tchaikovsky's *1812 Overture,* open every cabinet door, put a big trash can in the middle of the room, and just as the cannons are knockin' the heck out of Napoleon, throw out all of that crap you've been saving for company! The Russian Army is not coming to your house to celebrate; there's enough company on your hips.

You MUST keep the high-calorie, low-value foods out of your kitchen. And don't give them to the neighbors; they probably have pepperoni pizzas coming out the armpits. The Girl Scouts can still build campsites and plant trees if you buy their cookies and then flush them down the toilet. (You know, if the Girl Scouts really wanted to be "with it," they'd start selling sugar-free gum in the shape of little pup tents or something!)

A FINAL WORD ABOUT VOLUME (YOURS, THAT IS)

One pound of fat equals 3,500 calories. Some people can gain a pound a day. This means that they ate 3,500 MORE calories than their body needed. I know people who eat 3,500 calories in a single meal. Therefore, if you want to LOSE one pound of fat, you must deduct 3,500 calories from what your body needs for all of its normal activities. All you have to do is eat 500 fewer calories each day for a week and you'll lose that extra one or one and a half pounds.

Did you get that part?? One or one and a half pounds per week! I didn't just make up this number; it comes from medical evidence about human metabolism. If you lose weight any faster, you're just losing water and muscle tissue. The water comes back almost immediately, and losing muscle tissue can cause real physical problems. So when you hear somebody brag about losing ten pounds in one week, know that this person is not losing ten pounds of fat, and know that 90 percent of such a loss will return. The only way to lose fat is to lose it slowly. Listen to me because I have been there. I have gained and lost the weight of you and your wheelchair together. Take it slow and it will stay lost!

But the real key to the FOOD 4 LIFE plan is activity. Remember our activity formula on page 126? The people who can and should eat a fabulous dinner like the one you saw in Plan C are the ones who exercise every day and get to multiply their ideal weight by a factor of fifteen! The more active you are, the more food you get to eat and STILL lose weight! Let's say again that you want to lose 1 pound. In order to do that, you must consume 3,500 *fewer* calories than your body needs for regular maintenance. If you burn 300 or 400 extra calories each day in exercise, then those calories come right off the top of that magic 3,500. Burning 400 extra calories each day for a week will equal 2,800 lost calories. That's most of your weekly goal. You don't even have to have a calculator to get that score!

This is not a diet. A diet is a temporary food plan, and FOOD 4 LIFE is forever! (If we wanted temps, we'd go to Kelly Girl.) This way of life will make the pounds come off and stay off so that you can get busy with whatever else it is that you do best!

CHAPTER 5

EXERCISE and FOOD 4 LIFE: A Program for Children

Not long ago I received a letter from a woman with an incredible story. When her son was born, she was told that he had "multiple handicaps" and a condition called Down's syndrome. She was also told by a hospital staff physician that the "kindest" thing for her, the rest of her children, *and this child* would be to "let him die." She answered, "No."

Her letter continued, "In those early days, Richard, I felt that surely our son's disabilities were my punishment for past sins. I had stopped loving my husband; I resented my children for stealing my youth; when I was carrying this baby, I had wished that he had never been conceived. No one on Earth knew my evil thoughts. But God knew and I was sure that this was my message from Him that I could not be forgiven."

Several months later, she was told by the family physician that she should place her son in a residential facility. This way, he could receive the constant pro-fessional attention he would forever require. "And after all," the doctor told her, "you and your husband are almost fifty years old."

Again, she said, "No, he'll stay with our family."

I turned to the next page, and there, neatly stapled to the stationery was a beautiful family portrait. "And here's a picture of our family," she said, "at Mark's bar mitzvah. Mark *was* a message from God, but not a punishment. Rather, the message was that we could be a strong and healthy family again. It was Mark who showed us how; thank God I didn't let him die."

Maybe you've just had a doctor carefully and solemnly explain the specific ways that your baby will be "different." The feelings you are experiencing are like those of every other parent who's ever been in your place: "Why did this happen to *my* baby?" "Was it something that *I* did wrong, or, worse, something that I failed to do?"

You feel confused at first. You don't know whether or not this child will be a burden; you don't know what to do or where to turn. The first place to turn is to yourself. Know that you are a good person. This is not the wrath of God; it *just happened.* Your child's physical challenges are the result of very complex biological and chemical factors. These occurrences are nobody's fault! Destructive feelings like guilt, despair, rejection, and even overprotection will do *nothing* for your child now. And so no matter what you felt during those first few days or months, it's time to decide that your special, beautiful baby will grow to his or her complete potential.

But before I can convince you to teach your children exercise and good nutrition, I must first convince you to do it for yourself. If you are beginning our book at this point, go back and read the previous chapters on exercise and nutrition. Examine your own health habits. Start getting *your* body in shape and you can do the same thing for your child.

A child with physical challenges will take more time, more work, and more patience. You will curse and you will cry. But if you give him the chance, he will astonish you with what he can achieve and give. And if you give *yourself* a chance, you will become a much better and more meaningful human being.

AT WHAT AGE SHOULD YOUR CHILD BEGIN THE EXERCISE AND FOOD 4 LIFE PROGRAM?

The answer to this question depends entirely upon your child, his current physical condition, and the degree of his or her medical treatment. While the mental and physical development of ALL children follows some patterns, every child is different. And every family situation is different.

For example, many members of the Reach Foundation's advisory board felt that if you are the parent of an infant or a toddler with physical challenges you have enough to do just understanding and stabilizing your child's medical needs. On the other hand, you may be the parent of a three-year-old who should immediately begin a program of regular exercise.

This is a decision you must make with expert counseling. So study the EXERCISE 4 LIFE program, take this book to your doctor, and then decide.

There are two things upon which all experts agree:

1. A FAT child will have an additional and unnecessary disability.
2. A FAT child usually lives in a FAT household with FAT parents.

So even if your doctor feels that now is not the time for your child to exercise, begin the EXERCISE and FOOD 4 LIFE program *yourself.* That way you will be the best possible role-model when your child is ready.

Begin the EXERCISE 4 LIFE program by sharing the following letter with your son or daughter.

Richard Simmons
Los Angeles, CA

My Friend
Your Town, USA

Hi.

Before we begin your EXERCISE 4 LIFE program, I wanted to talk with you about "parts." You know, every body's got parts. Some parts work good most of the time, and some parts don't work at all. All parts are different that way.

Parts come in different numbers, different sizes, different colors, and different strengths. But none of these differences matters much. What matters is how each body uses the parts it's got.

So if an exercise mentions a part that you don't have—or a part that's not very strong right now—just ask your doctor how you can exercise one of your other parts. You could end up inventing a brand-new exercise—maybe even one that nobody in the entire world ever thought of before.

If you do, I'd love to hear all about it. Send me a description of your new exercise (and maybe a photograph or a drawing of yourself doing it). My address is:

Richard Simmons
The Reach Foundation
Orthopaedic Hospital
P.O. Box 60132, Terminal Annex
Los Angeles, California 90060

Love,

Richard Simmons

EXERCISE 4 LIFE: A Program for Children

The following exercises have been specially created just for you. You should try to do the entire program EVERY DAY. (It usually takes about an hour to complete.) As you improve, you'll probably want to do more, and when this happens, ask your doctor if you may select a few exercises from the adult program.

The therapists who have helped develop these exercises for the Reach Foundation are:

OrthopædicHospital

Consultants:

Patricia Davy-Schnall, R.P.T.
—Pediatric Clinical
    Coordinator

Vickie Cracchiolo, R.P.T.
—Staff Therapist

Lynne Morihisa, R.P.T.
—Staff Therapist

Lynn Lee, R.P.T.
—Assistant Director
    of Therapies

Jack Turman, R.P.T.
—Staff Therapist

Kim O'Brien, R.P.T.
—Staff Therapist

Orthopaedic Hospital
Los Angeles, CA

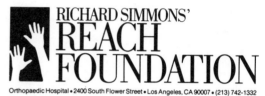

RICHARD SIMMONS' REACH FOUNDATION

Orthopaedic Hospital • 2400 South Flower Street • Los Angeles, CA 90007 • (213) 742-1332

Consultant:

Tim Green
—Exercise Coordinator
Reach Foundation
Los Angeles, CA

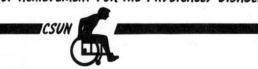

CENTER OF ACHIEVEMENT FOR THE PHYSICALLY DISABLED

CSUN

CAL STATE UNIVERSITY NORTHRIDGE
Physical Education Department

18111 Nordhoff St.
Northridge, California 91330

Consultant:

Sam Britten, Ph.D.
—Director
Center of Achievement for the Physically Disabled
California State University, Northridge
Northridge, CA

THE MODELS APPEARING IN THIS CHAPTER ARE:

Arthur (age 6),
a child with Duchenne muscular dystrophy.

Axel (age 12),
a child with postpolio.

Jeffery (age 14),
a child with spina bifida.

Karen (age 4),
a child with Christmas Disease (a form of hemophilia).

Kathryn (age 6),
a child with spina bifida.

Narayana (age 9),
a child with bilateral below-knee amputation.

Quinten (age 8),
a child with spina bifida.

Stephanie (age 8),
a child with Christmas Disease and lupus.

Rene (age 10),
a child with spina bifida.

IMPORTANT NOTE: If this is the first section you are reading, please turn to pages 22-23 for a short lesson in breathing techniques. (It's real important, honest!)

If you've already looked at our exercises for adults, you'll notice that we have a slightly different format here. The first three exercises in our children's program emphasize breathing and stretching. Use them to get your body ready for the more active work-out that completes the chapter. And we have excluded isometric and isotonic movements since they may be a little advanced for some kids.

In some of the exercises you'll see the phrase "repeat as able." This simply means that you should recognize your own individual needs and abilities. If one repetition is all you can do at first, then one is better than none. Begin slowly and add repetitions as needed. If you can do as many as ten repetitions, then you should ask your doctor about adding additional exercises from the adult section.

Finally, if you're in a wheelchair, be sure to lock the wheels and fasten your seat belt!!

CWU1   Blow the Boat

Position: standing, sitting, or lying on back.

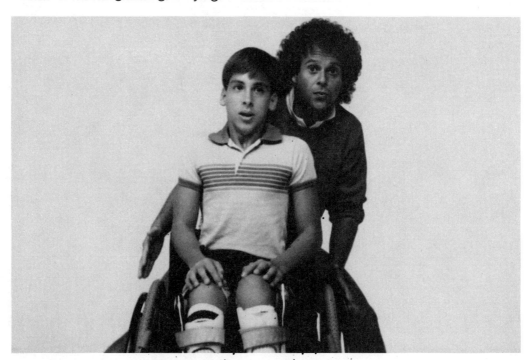

1. Straighten your back, just like Jeffery is doing.

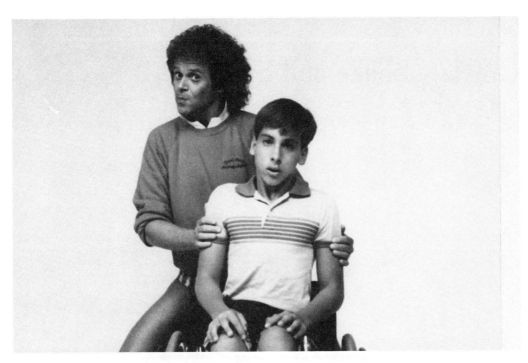

2. Take a deep breath. Pull in your stomach as much as you can and hold for five seconds.

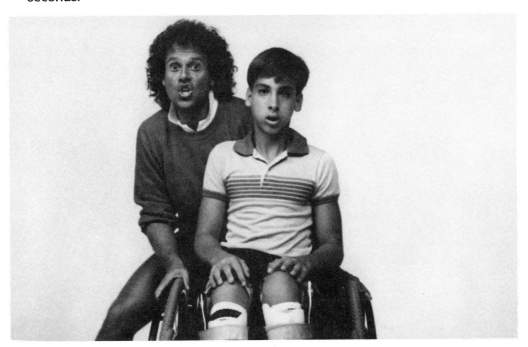

3. Pretend you're blowing a sailboat across the ocean. Slowly release your breath, sticking your stomach out as far as you can. Keep blowing, as long as you can.

4. Breathe! Breathe! (Whew, that was close!)

CWU2   Shake and Stop

Position: lying on back.

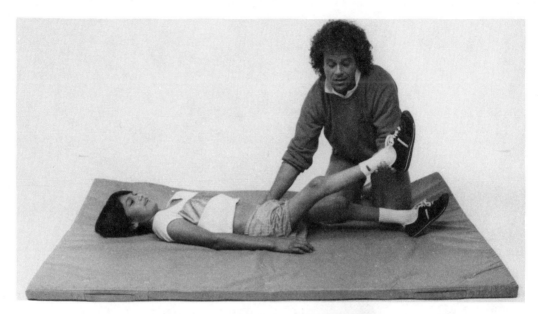

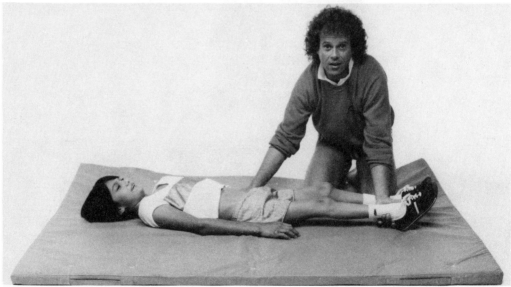

1. Briskly shake right leg, the same way Axel is doing. Stop and hold leg perfectly still.

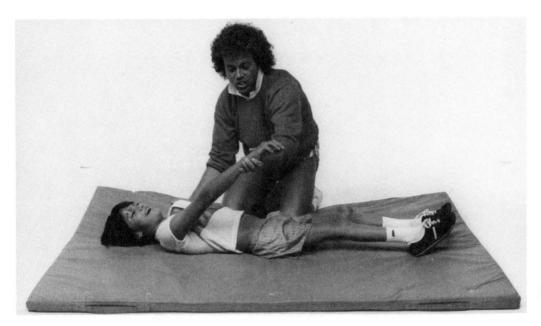

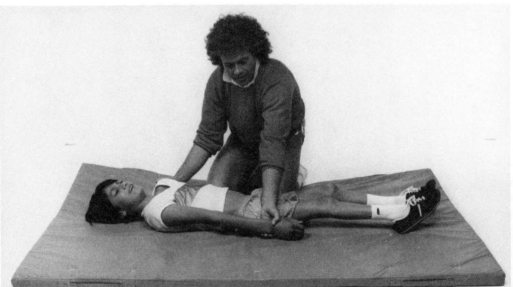

2. Briskly shake right arm. Stop and hold arm perfectly still.
3. Alternate sides and repeat exercise first with left leg and then left arm.
4. Pretend you're a milk shake and briskly shake your entire body. Stop and hold perfectly still.

Note: This exercise helps you learn how first to relax and then move your muscles on command.

CWU3   Lazy Bones

Position: standing, sitting, or lying on back.

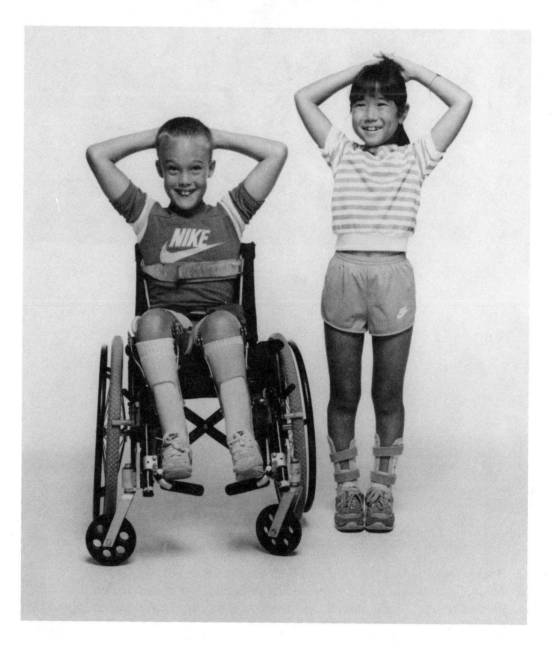

1. Interlock your fingers behind your head, just like Quinten and Stephanie are doing.

2. Now slowly stretch back as far as you can.
3. Don't fall over—but yawn and move that stretch all over your front. It feels so good!

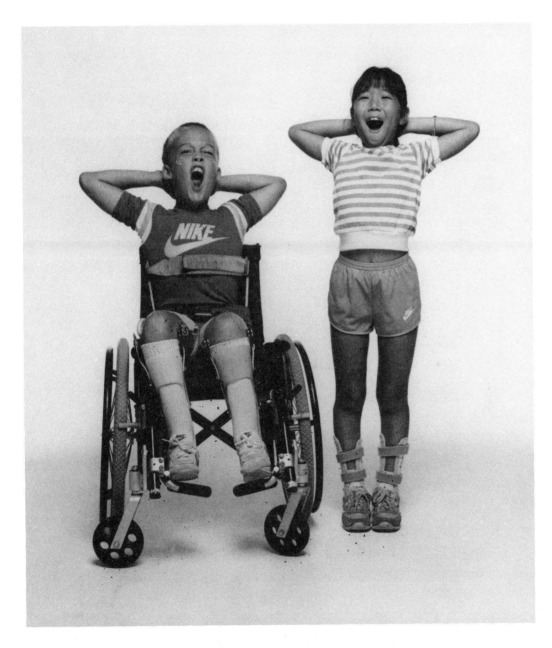

Note: Most of us sit all day, leaning forward. This exercise helps us stretch out the muscles in our middles and helps with good posture.

FACE

CFA1 Happy Face

Position: standing, sitting, or lying on back.

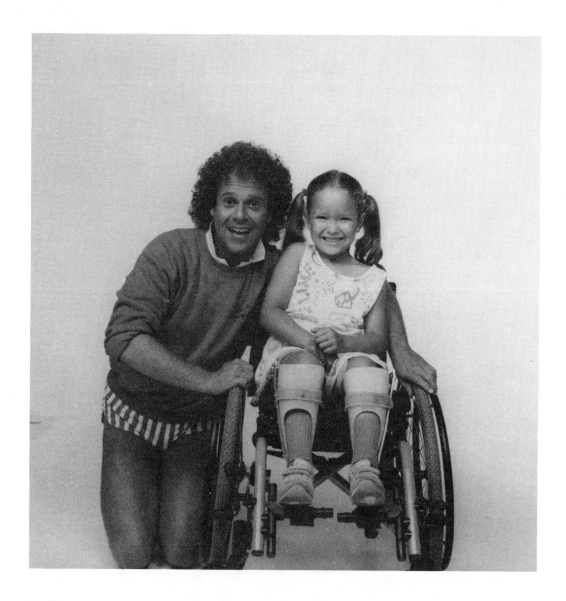

1. Show a happy face like Kathryn's by making a great big smile.

Note: Faces need exercise, too, 'cause they help us communicate with people.

CFA2 Mad Face

Position: standing, sitting, or lying on back.

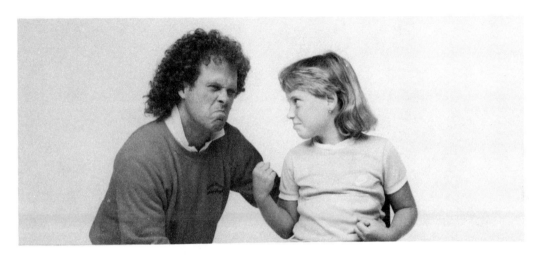

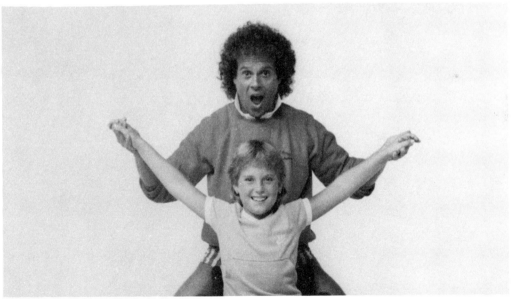

1. Everybody, even somebody *very* nice, gets mad sometimes. Show your mad face by tightening your lips and wrinkling your forehead.

    Now give me a Happy Face again, 'cause Rene and I were just pretending to be mad!

NECK

CN1   Elephant Trunk Swings

Position: standing, sitting, or lying on back, arms at sides.

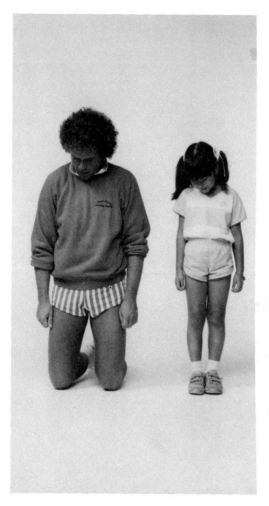 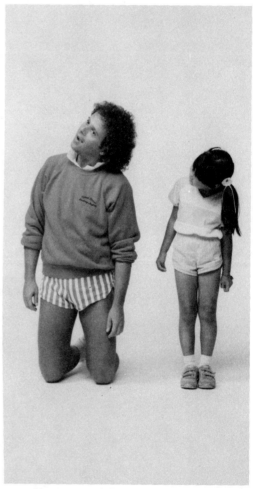

1. Bend your had slightly forward, just like Karen and me.
2. Sway your head to your right shoulder.

3. Sway your head to your left shoulder.

4. Continue these two movements as you sway your head slowly, just like an elephant sways his trunk.

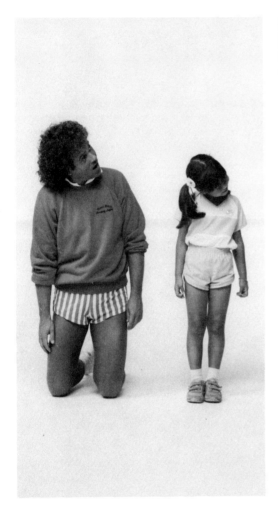 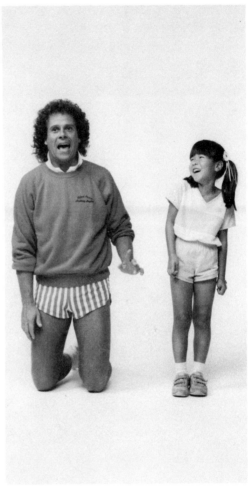

5. Now pretend the elephant is taking a shower by squirting water all over himself. (Karen thinks that's silly!)

Note: This is a great exercise for releasing tension in your neck and shoulders.

CN2   Nodding

Position: standing, sitting, or lying on back.

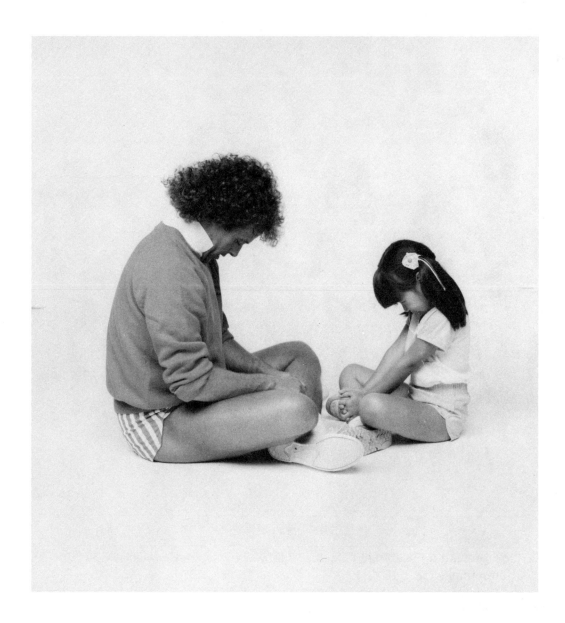

1. Bring head forward so that your chin rests on your chest.

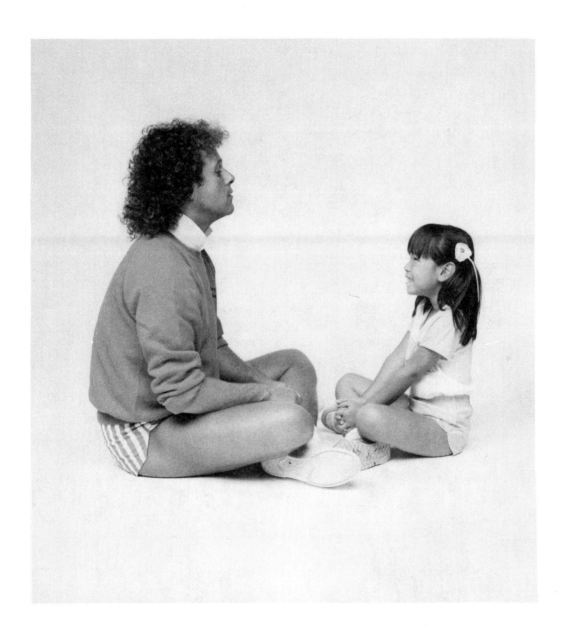

2. Now lift head up so that you are looking straight ahead.
3. Return chin to chest and repeat as able.

SHOULDERS AND ARMS _____
CSH1 "I Don't Know"

Position: standing, sitting, or lying on back.

1. Keeping back straight, shrug shoulders.

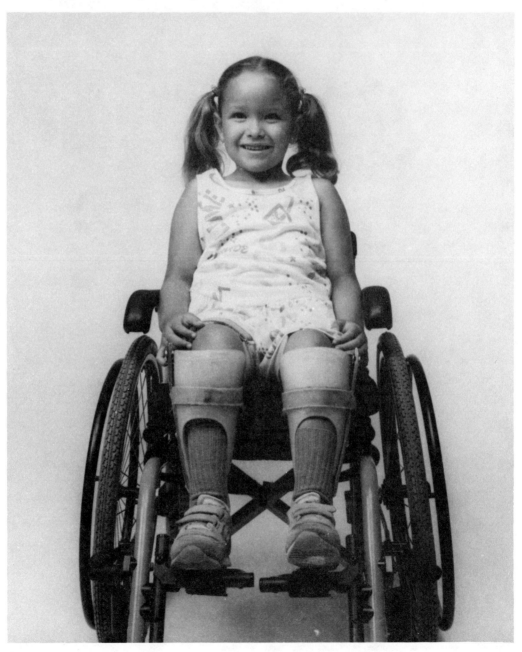

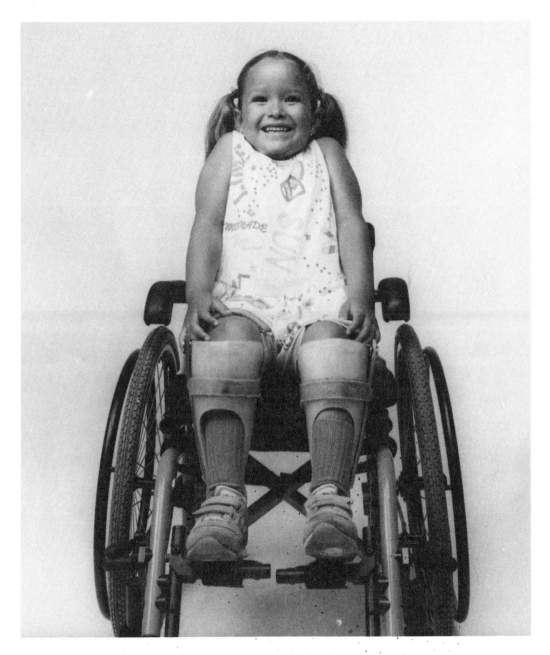

2. Now really push shoulders back and try to pinch your shoulder blades together.
3. Relax shoulders and repeat as able.

Note: This is a good one to practice when your mom asks who got into the peanut butter. It also strengthens the muscles in your shoulders and upper back and helps with good posture.

CSH2 Train Choo-Choos

Position: standing or sitting, arms at sides.

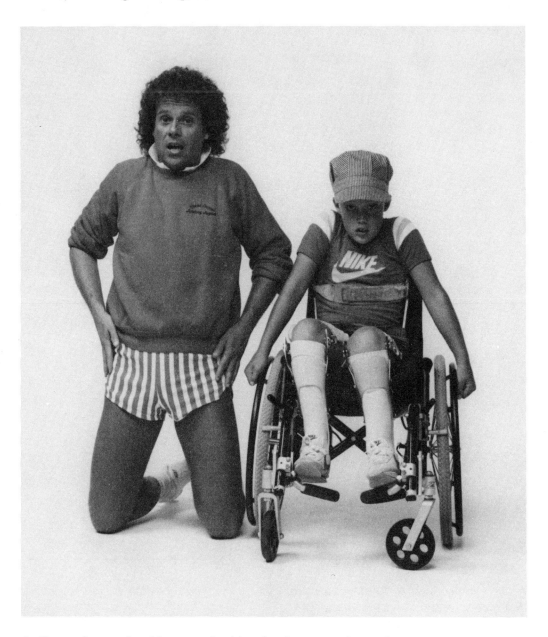

1. Pretend your shoulders are the big wheels on a train engine.
2. Keeping arms at sides, move shoulders in a smooth, continuous circle: first up, then forward, then down, and then back.

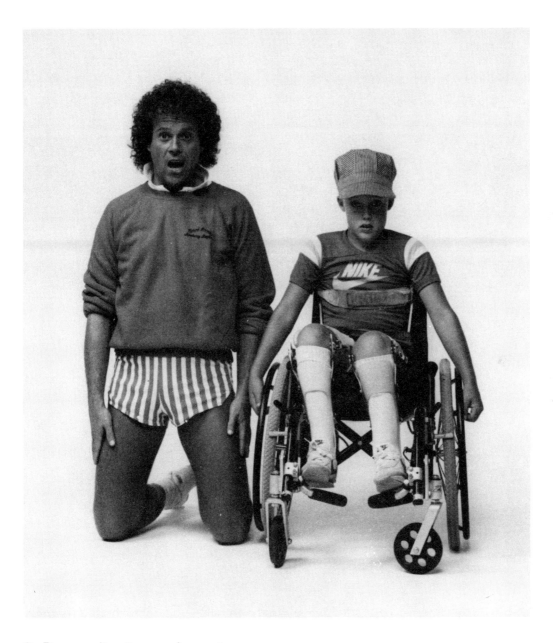

3. Reverse directions and repeat.
    Choo-Choo! Chugga! Chugga! Chugga!

CSH3   Superkid

Position: lying on stomach.

1. Straighten your arms out overhead, in the same way as Arthur.

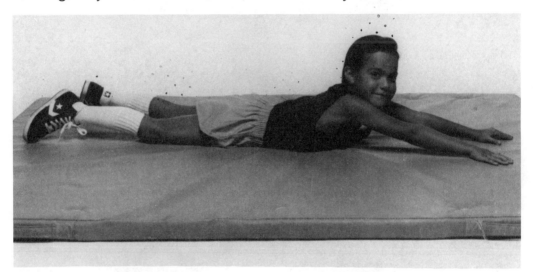

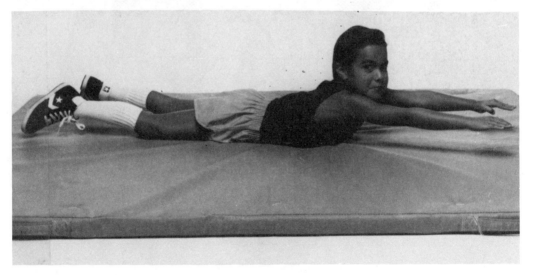

2. Keeping elbows straight, lift head and arms as far as you can without discomfort. Hold for five seconds.
3. Pretend you're flying all over your neighborhood.

Note: It's okay if your feet come up just a little, but try to keep them down.

CSH4   Catch the Bug

Position: standing, sitting, or lying on back.

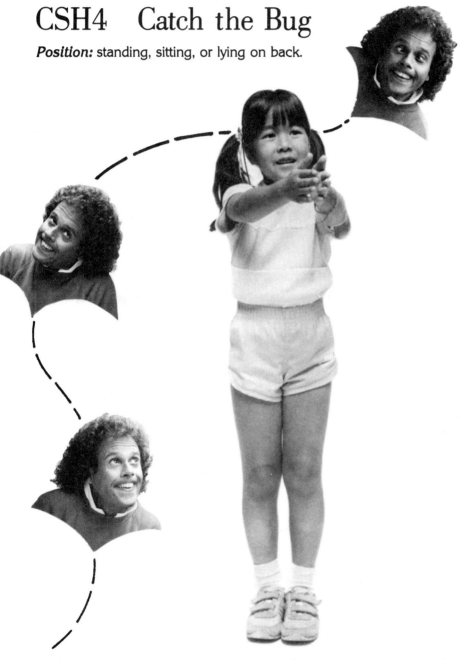

1. Pretend that a pesky little bug is flying all around your head. (Richard's pretending to be a bug for Karen.)
2. Keeping your elbows straight, slap your hands together at all the places it might fly.
3. It's very fast, so you may not get it at first. Keep trying!

CSH5   Helicopter

Position: standing or sitting.

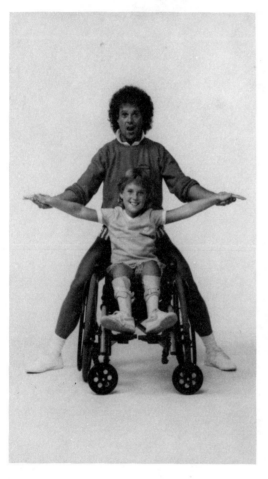 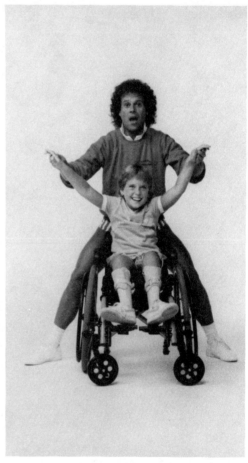

1. Keeping elbows straight, stretch arms out to sides.
2. Pretend that you're a helicopter and your arms are rotor blades. Start your engines by making tiny little circles with your arms.

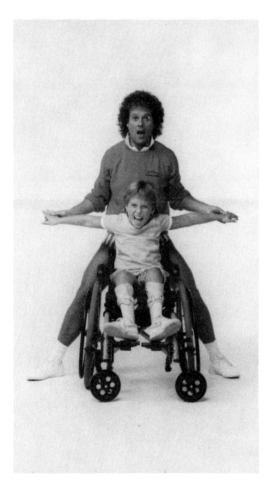 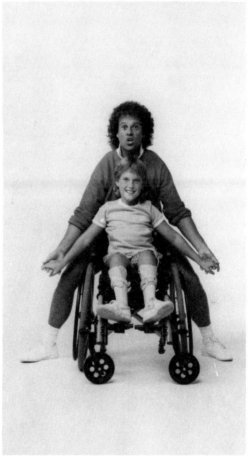

3. It's lift-off, so move your arms in bigger circles. Now make the biggest circles you can as you hit "turbo-boost."

4. Slow your engines and come in for a landing.

Note: This one's more fun if you also make swishing sounds.

It helps strengthen your back muscles and is especially good if you've been sitting in a chair all day.

CSH6   Armchair Push-Ups

Position: sitting in a chair (or a wheelchair) that has armrests.

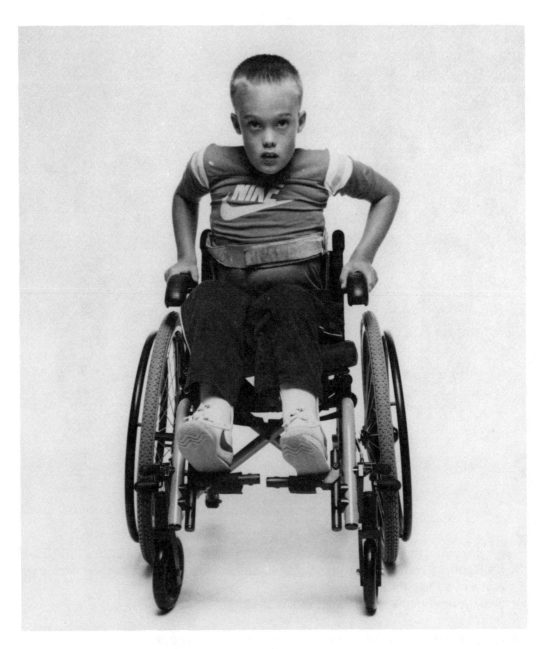

1. Put your hands on chair armrests or the rims of your wheelchair (or even the seat of the chair).

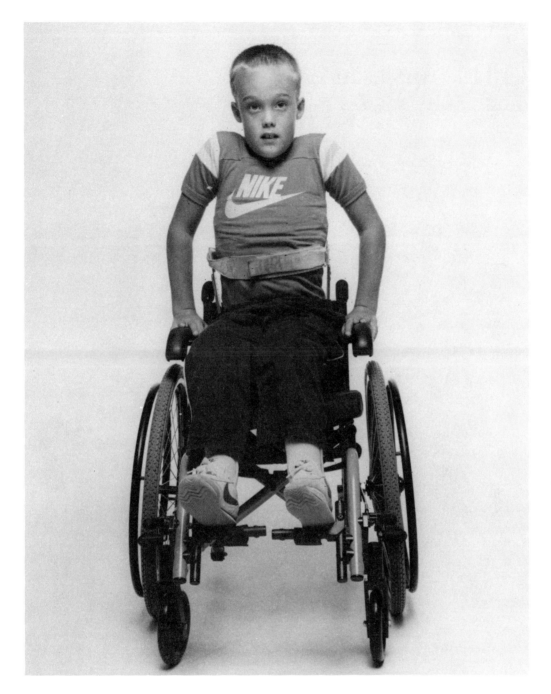

2. Push down as you straighten your elbows and raise your bottom off the seat. Hold for five seconds.

3. Return to starting position and repeat as able.

Note: This exercise can strengthen the muscles in your upper arms. It can also keep your bottom from getting sore if you've been sitting too long.

FINGERS

CFI1   Applesauce

Position: standing, sitting, or lying on back.

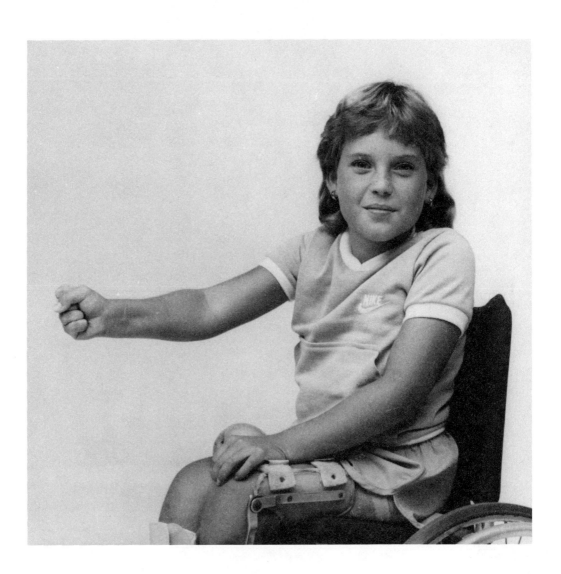

1. Make a fist around an imaginary apple.

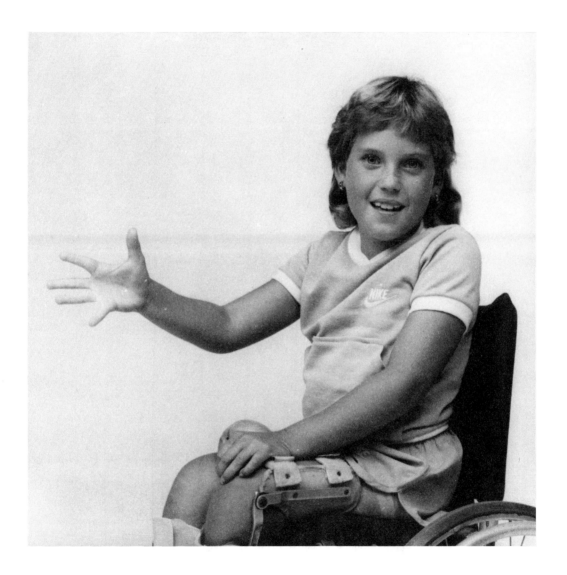

2. Squeeze your hand and pretend you're making applesauce. Now open your hand and repeat as able.

3. Alternate hands and repeat as able.

Note: This one will help you squeeze that toothpaste tube every morning!

CFI2 Walking Fingers

Position: standing, sitting, or lying on back, near a flat surface like a table, countertop, or book. You can even use your thigh, just like Axel.

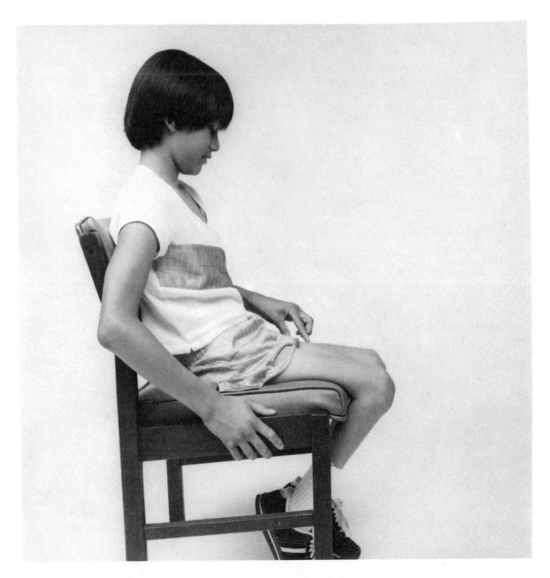

1. Use two fingers to walk across the flat surface. First use your thumb and index finger. Then use your index and second finger and so on until you have used all your fingers.
2. Alternate hands and repeat as able.
3. Now walk all fingers and pretend you're a funny, ten-legged spider.

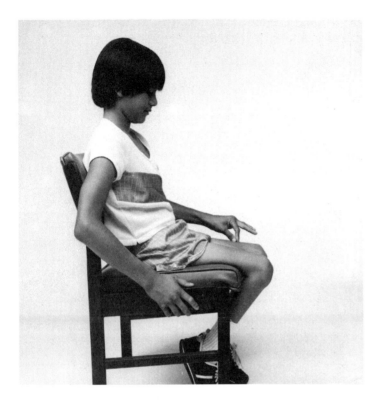

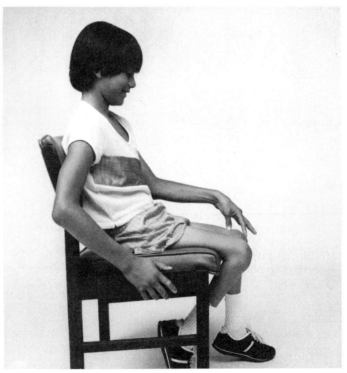

WRIST
CWR   Hello and Goodbye

Position: standing, sitting, or lying on back.

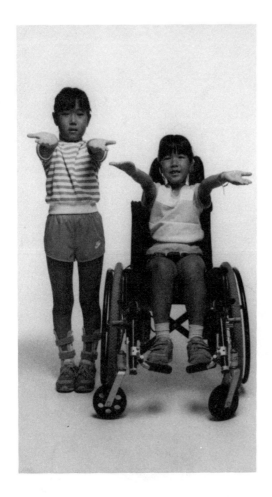 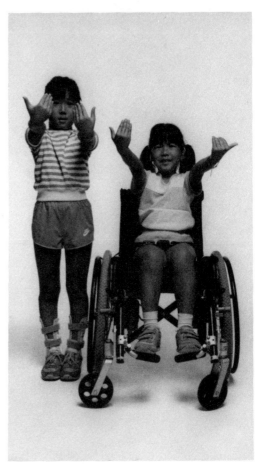

1. Stretch your arms (palms up) in front of your body.
2. Keeping your elbows straight, bend your wrists toward your body. Wave hello to yourself.

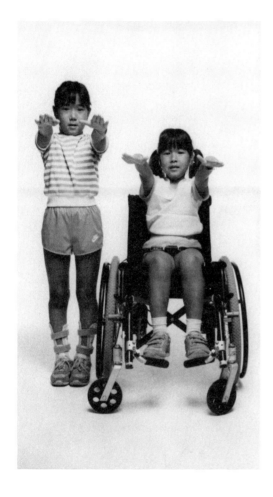
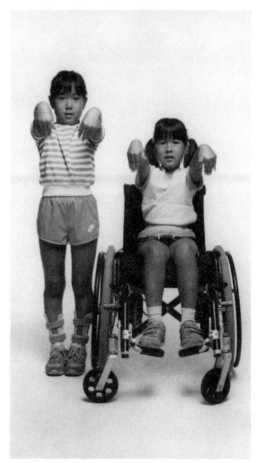

3. Return to starting position and repeat as able.
4. Now turn your palms down and wave goodbye to someone else.
5. Return to starting position and repeat as able.

Note: This exercise helps give your wrist the flexibility you need when you're dressing yourself or doing Hawaiian hand language.
    P.S. Did you notice that Stephanie and Karen are sisters?

ELBOW

CEL   Row, Row, Row Your Boat

Position: standing, sitting, or lying on back.

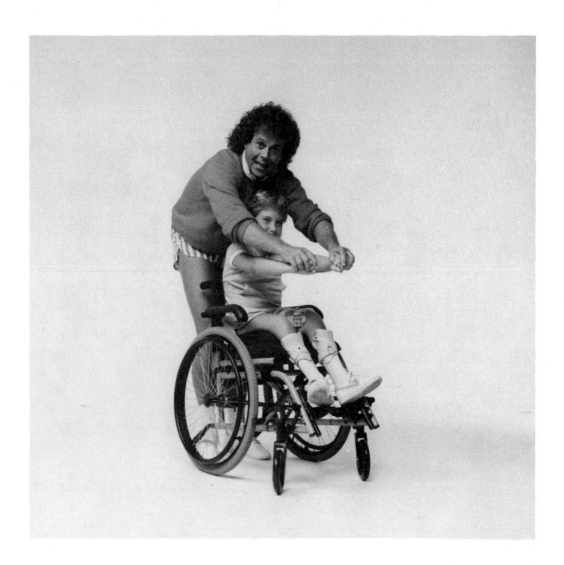

1. Stretch arms in front of body.

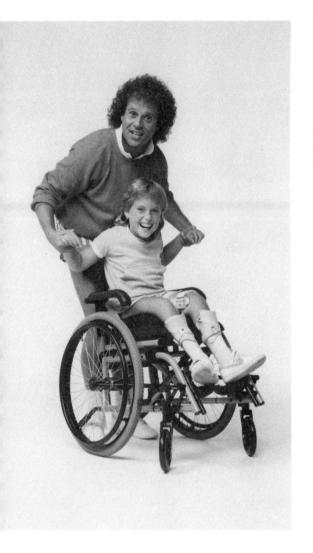
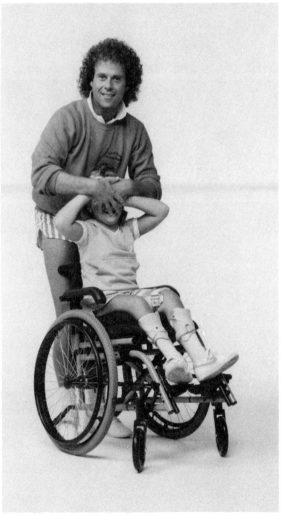

2. Bend elbows and bring arms back and to the side.
3. Now straighten elbows as you stretch arms forward again. Repeat as able.

Oh my goodness! Rene's boat just hit the dock!

WAIST AND STOMACH
CWS1   Soaring

Position: sitting in a chair (if in wheelchair, be sure to lock the wheels and fasten the seat belt).

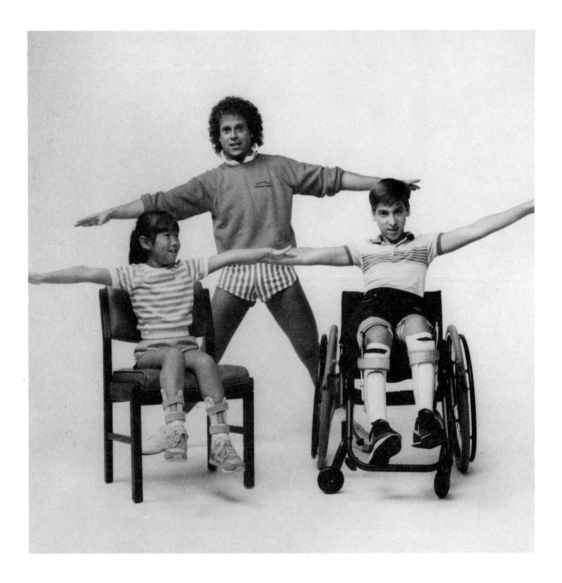

1. Keeping elbows straight, stretch arms out to side.

2. Bending at waist, lean to the left and try to touch the floor.
3. Return to first step and then lean to the right. Repeat as able.

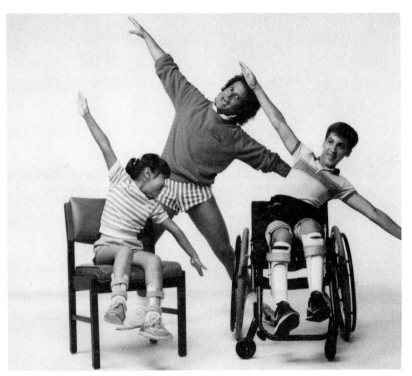

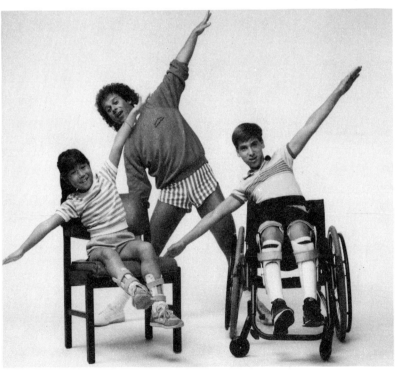

CWS2   Tummy Twist

Position: standing with feet apart or sitting.

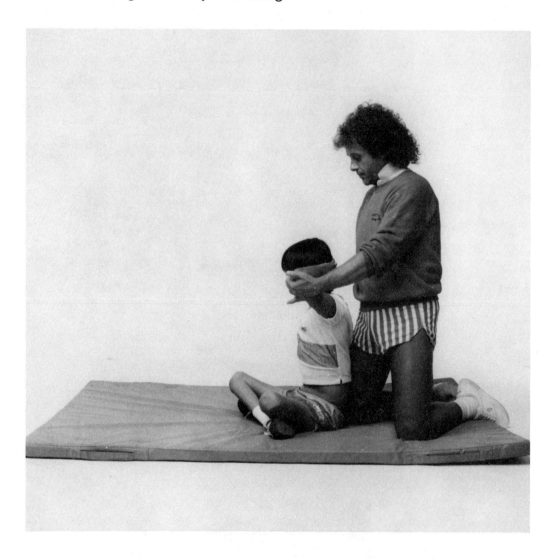

1. Keeping back straight, put hands behind head.

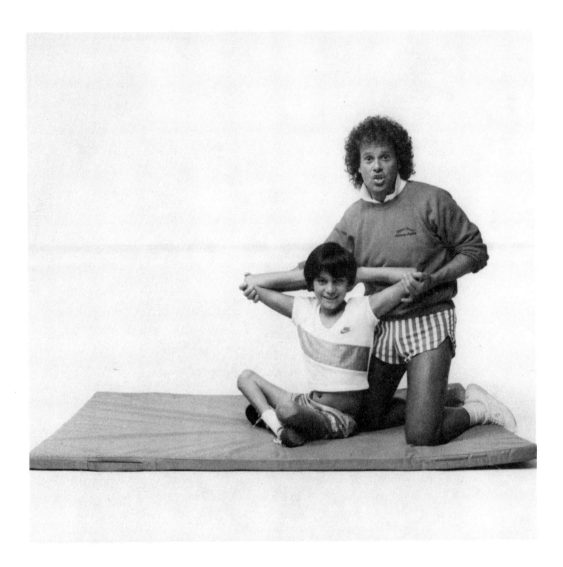

2. Keeping hips and legs still, turn body to the left. (Remember, we want a big exhale as you move!)

3. Return to starting position, and turn body to the right.

4. Repeat as able.

Note: Now you're also stretching the muscles that help you to turn and reach over your shoulder.

CWS3   Your Majesty

Position: standing or sitting (if in a wheelchair, fasten seat belt and lock wheels).

1. Straighten arms (palms down) in front of chest.

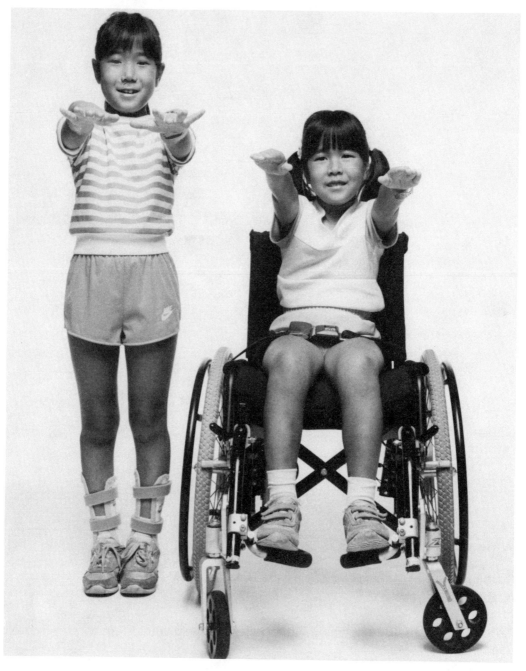

2. Bending forward at waist, reach for the floor.
3. Return to starting position and repeat as able.

Note: If sitting, try to touch head to knees. If standing, you may want to bend your knees a little. Once you make it down there, you get to scratch your toes.

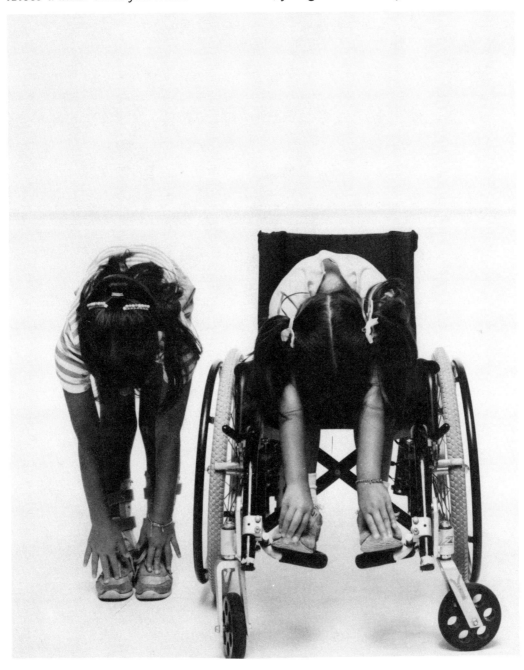

CWS4 Curl-Ups

Position: lying on back, legs straight.

1. Keeping arms straight, curl your head and shoulders and reach toward your knees.
2. Slowly lower to starting position and repeat as able.

Note: Be careful not to strain your neck muscles—let your stomach do the work!

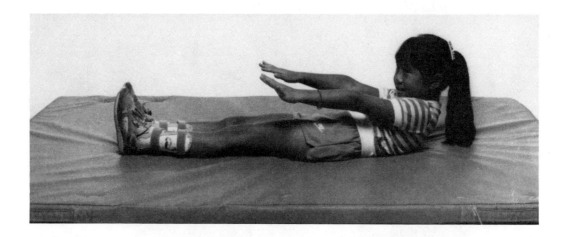

Variation: When you can do this easily, put your hands across your chest and repeat as able. When you get *really* good at this, put your hands behind your head and repeat as able.

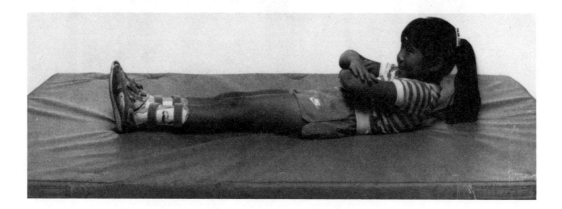

CWS5   Airplane

Position: lying on stomach.

1. I don't think you've met Narayana yet. With palms down, lift arms up in the air and slightly away from sides, just as he is doing.
2. Raise your chest off the floor.
3. Return to starting position and repeat as able.

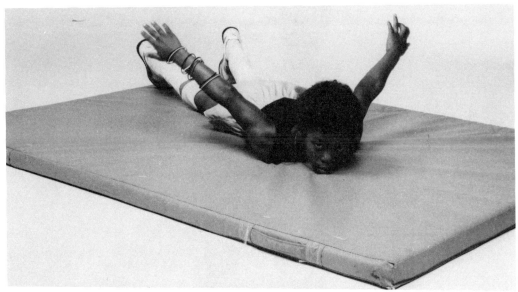

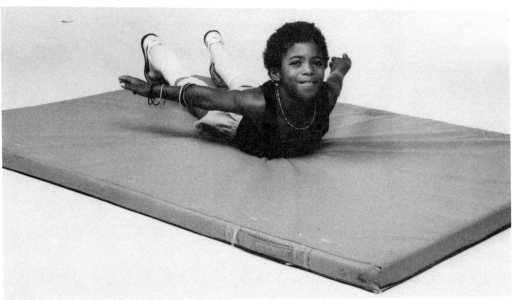

CWS6 Pelvic Tilt

Position: sitting in chair.

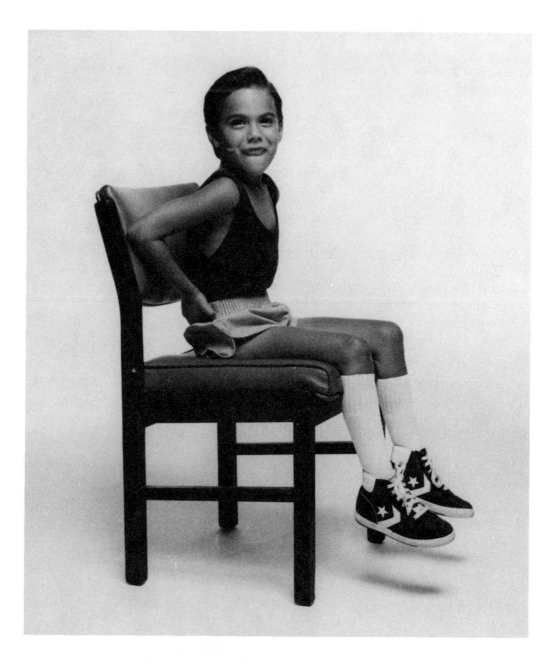

1. Put your hands in the small of your back.

2. Now try to flatten out the curve in your spine by shifting your hips backward.

Note: Pulling in your stomach muscles will help.

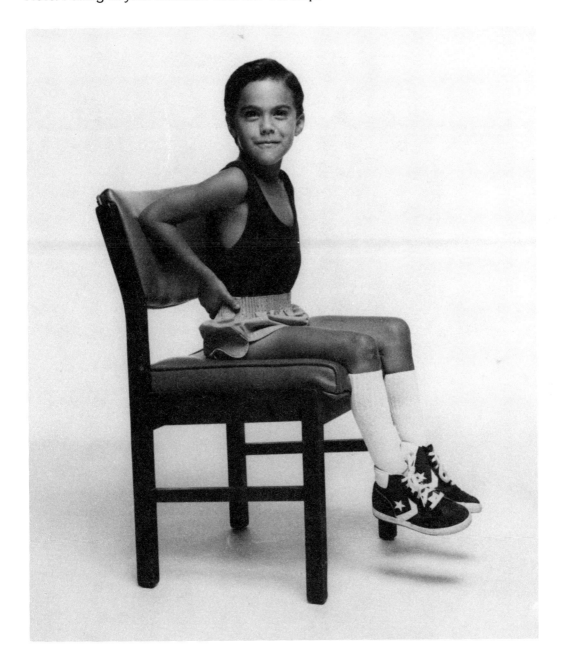

Variation: You can get the same effect by bringing your knees to your chest.

HIPS AND BUTTOCKS
CHB1   Marching in Place

Position: sitting in chair.

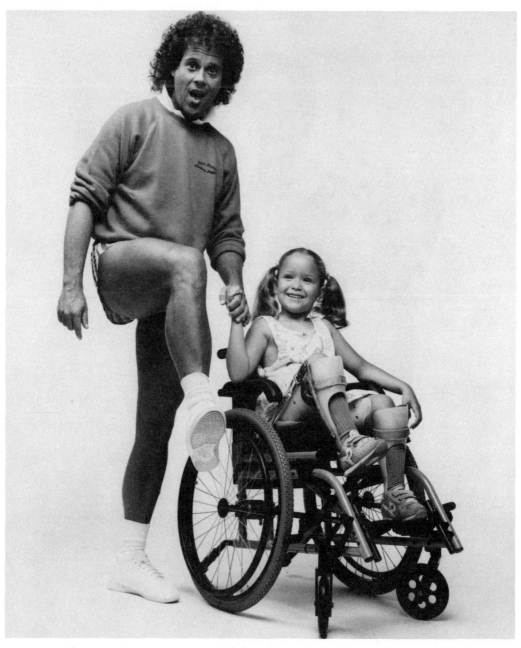

1. Sit up as straight as you can.
2. Lift knees one at a time and pretend you're marching in a parade.

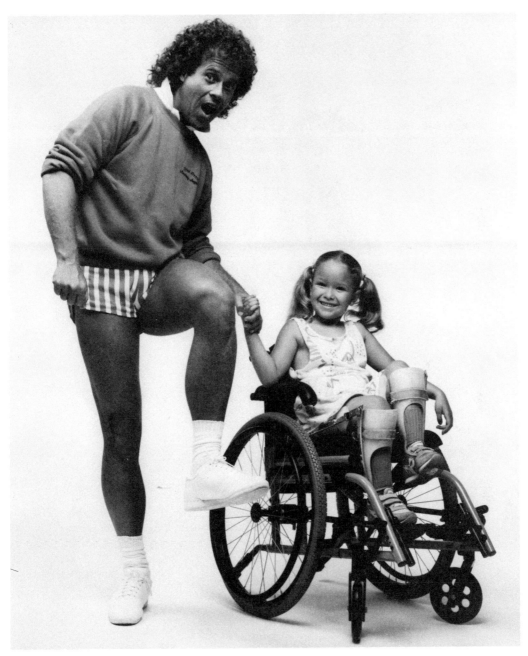

Note: This exercise helps strengthen the muscles you use when you put on a pair of jeans.

CHB2   Kick-Ups

Position: standing behind a chair, holding on to chairback.

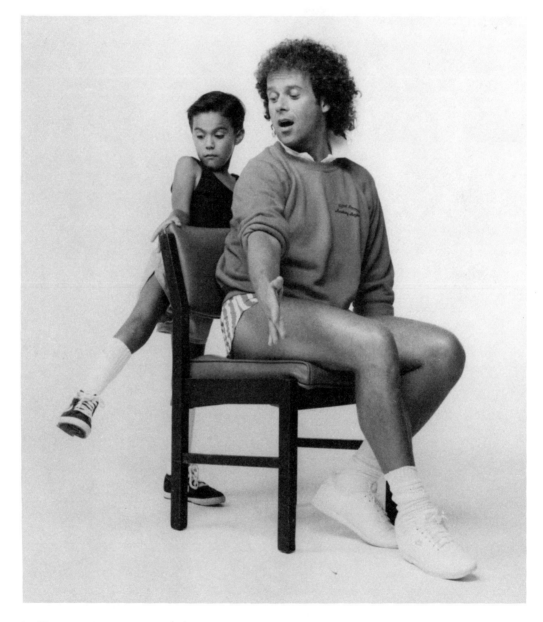

1. Keeping knee as straight as possible, lift right leg sideward as far as you can without discomfort. (Be sure to keep your trunk erect and not let it rotate or tilt to the side.) Return to starting position.

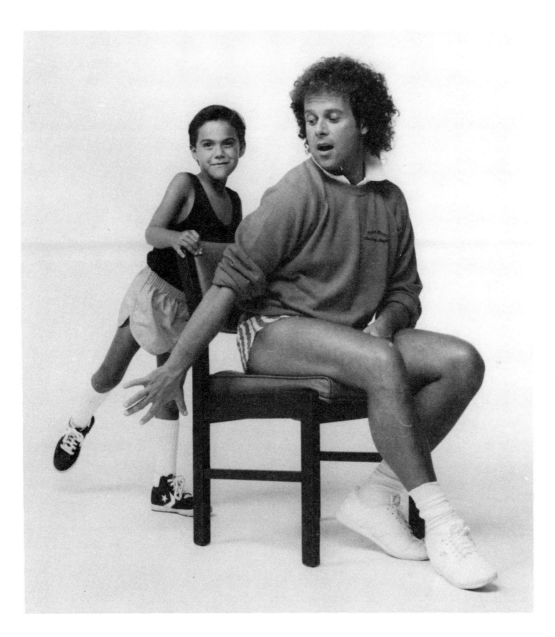

2. Now lift leg backward and return.
3. Alternate legs and repeat as able.

CHB3   Sitting Like a Diamond

Position: sitting on floor.

1. Bend knees and put soles of feet together. Your legs are in the shape of a diamond.

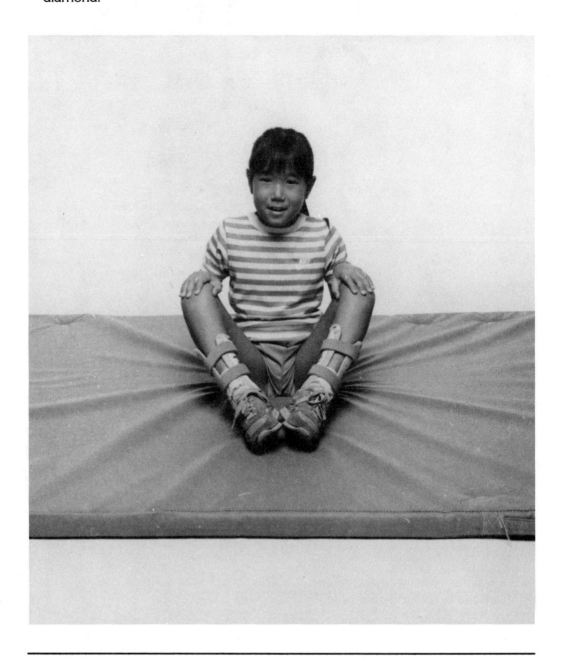

2. Placing hands on the insides of knees, try to push knees to floor. Continue until you feel a slight pull on your inner thighs. Don't push too hard!

3. Return to starting position and repeat as able.

Note: Sitting for long periods of time can make these muscles very stiff. This exercise helps keep them flexible so that you can more easily dress yourself and use the bathroom.

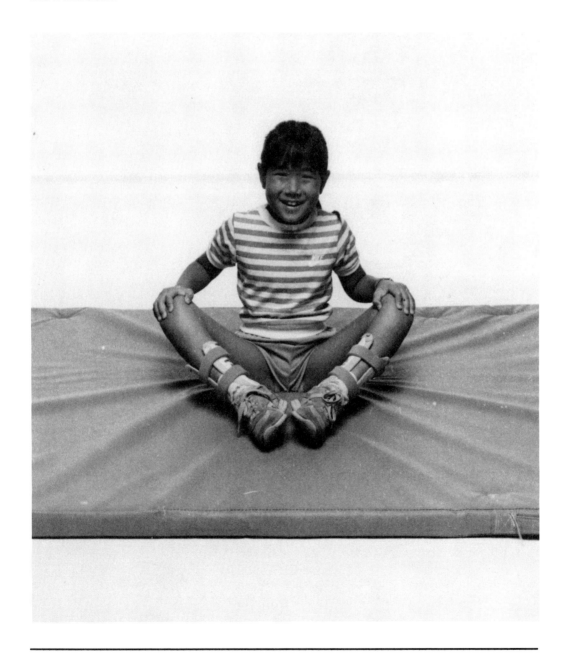

KNEES
CK1 Soccer Kicks

Position: sitting in chair.

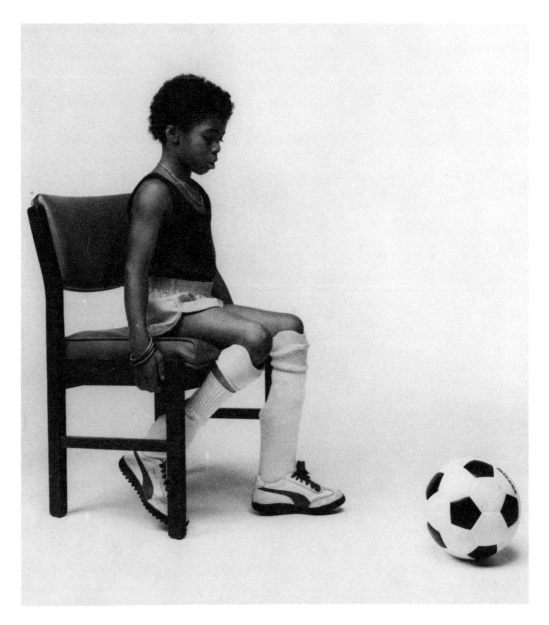

1. Sit upright with knees bent.
2. Now bring right leg as far back under your chair as you can.

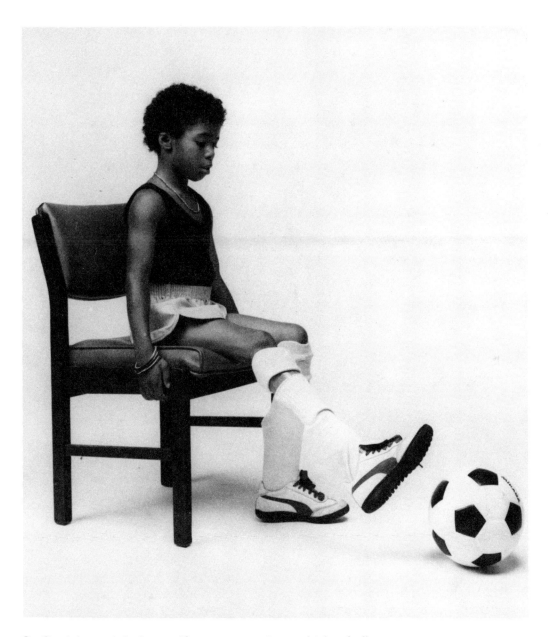

3. Straighten right leg as if you were going to kick a ball.
4. Relax and return to starting position.
5. Alternate legs and repeat as able.

CK2   Kick Your Bottom

Position: lying on stomach.

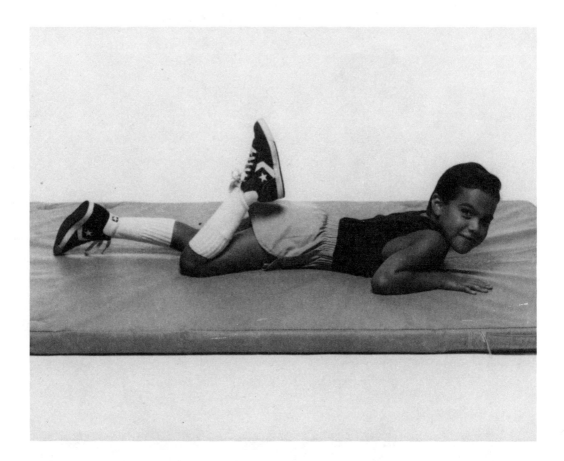

1. Bend right knee back so that ankle touches your bottom. (Well, maybe it *almost* touches your bottom. Keep trying!)
2. Return to starting position and repeat.
3. Alternate and repeat as able.

ANKLE

CAK1   Sock Hop

Position: sitting in chair, knees and feet together.

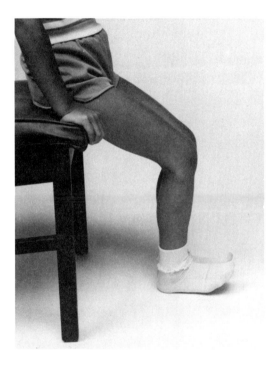

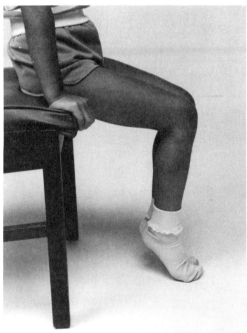

1. Keeping heels on floor (or on the footrest of your wheelchair), lift toes and feet to ceiling.
2. Reverse by keeping toes on floor and lifting heels to ceiling.

Note: You may need to work real hard at keeping your knees together.
This exercise keeps your feet flexible so your shoes'll fit better.

CAK2   Ankle Circles

Position: sitting in chair.

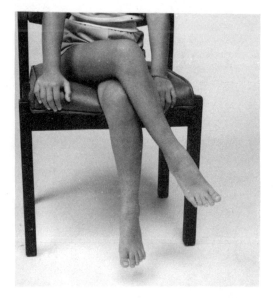

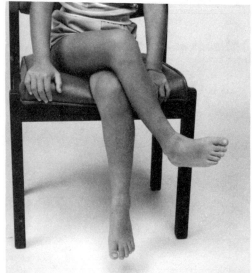

1. Cross your right leg over your left knee.
2. Move your right foot in a big circle (clockwise direction).

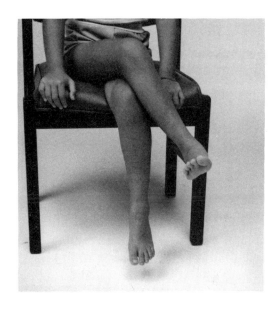

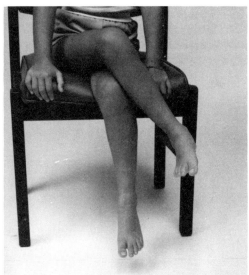

3. Reverse direction and roll foot counterclockwise.
4. Now cross your left leg over your right knee and repeat as able.

TOES

CT   Toe Wiggles

Position: sitting (shoes off).

1. Pretend your toes are wiggle worms. They want to squirm and look around.

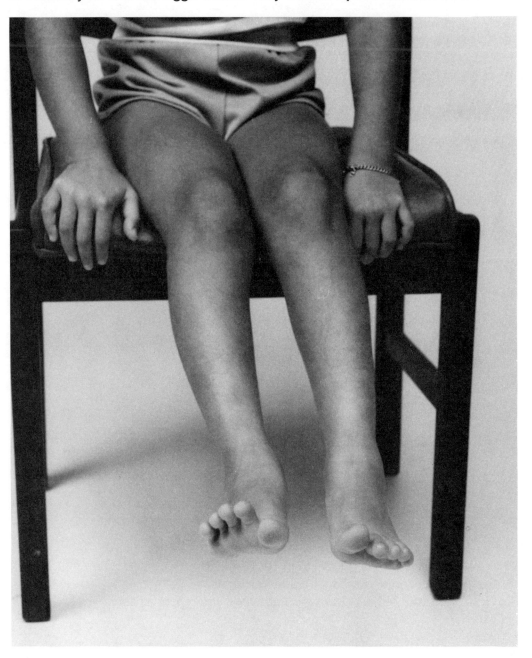

2. Move your toes up and down and all around, any way they want to go.

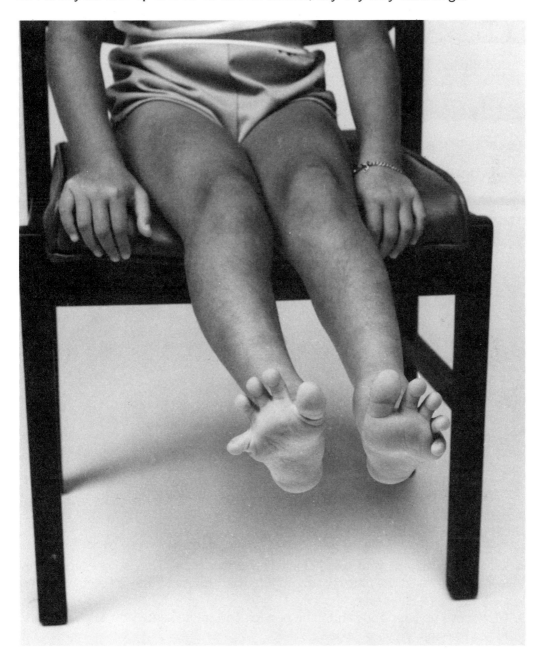

COOL-DOWN

Repeat the warm-up exercises (Blow the Boat, Shake and Stop, and Lazy Bones) and then follow them with this special relaxation exercise.

CCD Sleepy Parts

Position: relaxing in a comfortable position. (You can even grin if you feel like it!)

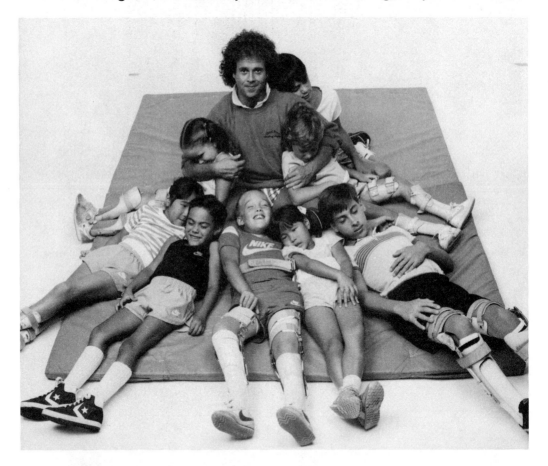

1. The work of this exercise is done with your brain.
2. Let your mind visit your toes. Think only about them. Concentrate upon how calm and relaxed they are. Slowly wiggle each toe until they all feel calm and sleepy.
3. Now move up your body and think of each part in the same way. The next parts to put to sleep are your ankles.

4. Continue using your brain to put your body parts to sleep: knees, thighs, fingers, hands, forearms, elbows, upper arms, hips, stomach, chest, neck, face, and head (don't forget your ears—they need to relax, too).

You've done a super job today. It wasn't easy, but you worked hard and your body's gonna love you for it. I'm very, very proud of you!

FOOD 4 LIFE: FOR PARENTS

The *best* thing you can do to improve your child's eating habits is to improve your own! So if you haven't read it yet, turn to Chapter Four, FOOD 4 LIFE. Good nutrition is good nutrition, no matter what your age. Growing children need regular and balanced portions of all nutrients, so begin your child's FOOD 4 LIFE program by talking to a doctor or registered dietitian. If your child has special nutritional requirements, the doctor or dietitian can coordinate those needs with our food plan. Otherwise, start your entire family on this program today! Remember, four-year-olds do not buy their own candy bars, ice cream, and pretzels! And by the time your child is old enough to select his own food, he will be influenced by the food habits *you've* established.

If your child is fat, it's your fault. And don't try making excuses about grandparents, Easter baskets, and birthday cake. A few sweets on holidays won't kill anybody. It's chips at every lunch, dessert at every meal, and bedtime snacks that make your child fat. Even if you do have a problem communicating this to grandparents, *you* must be the one to educate them about your child's needs. Start by having them read the following letter:

Dear Loving Grandparents,

I know that you love your grandchild more than life itself. I know that when you heard the news about his physical challenges the pain was so great that you died a little inside.

You'd do <u>anything</u> to help, but usually all you can do is stand and watch. So when you see that precious grandchild of yours, you give him one of your special brownies 'cause that always makes him smile. And after all, isn't it a grandparent's job to spoil grandchildren?

But brownies aren't the answer. They may make <u>you</u> feel better, but they can be poison for this child. Because of the physical challenges, your grandson or granddaughter probably gets less exercise and needs fewer calories than other kids. Extra calories mean fat. And fat means that his movements are even more difficult and his challenges even greater.

Give hugs and kisses instead of brownies. Talk and listen and share with him all of the wonderful things you know this life can offer. That's how you can help, 'cause, like all kids, he's got a lot to learn.

Love,

Richard Simmons

FOOD 4 LIFE: FOR KIDS

Your body is a fantastic machine. Every day it turns food and water into the energy necessary to run the whole system. Everything from thinking to moving needs this food and water fuel. Your body even has a way of saving extra fuel just in case you ever get stranded on a raft in the ocean and can't find anything for lunch. It does this by manufacturing fat and storing it in some of the "out of the way" and "unused" parts of your body. You've seen fat on meat or chicken? Well, the fat stored on your body is just the same. You can probably find your fat storage areas pretty easily—around your middle, on the tops of your legs, or on your bottom. The trouble comes when your body starts storing too much fat and you don't take that trip on the raft. Pretty soon all of your extra fuel supplies start getting in the way of other things your body wants to do. Simple things you used to do all the time become difficult when you have lots of extra fat.

You might be able to adapt to that, but if you already have extra fat, you know something else about it. Other kids make fun of it. If your name is Stewart, they start calling you "Stew-Pot," or they call you "Lardy" when you've told them a thousand times your name is Laurie. You know that some kids just don't know any better, but it still hurts.

The very best thing about this body of yours is that you can control the amount of fat it stores. You do this by controlling what you eat. Many years ago, some very smart doctors and nutritionists thought of a way to help you remember which foods make the most fat and which foods give you lots of energy with only a little fat.

All you have to do is think of a traffic signal. Each light on the signal has a special meaning: Red means stop, yellow means caution, and green means go.

Red foods are more easily turned into fat, and so your body needs fewer of these. Examples include cake, candy, cookies, ice cream, cheese, red meats, nuts, avocados, peanut butter, eggs, sweet potatoes, butter, soft drinks, chips, pretzels, olives, sugary cereals, and all desserts. You should eat red foods only once or twice a week, and even then in small amounts.

Eat yellow foods with caution. Much of your diet will come from this group, but your body works best with only a few daily servings of yellow food. Yellow foods include milk, creamy soups, turkey, popcorn, tuna, fruits, fruit juices, tortillas, peas, chicken, diet drinks, potatoes, corn, beans, nonsugared cereals, fish, bread, low-fat cheese, beans, and rice.

Green foods mean go. You can eat them at any time you feel hungry. They include green vegetables (like cucumbers, green beans, lettuce, broccoli, brussels sprouts, asparagus, celery), other vegetables (like cauliflower, squash, and carrots), tomatoes, vegetable juice, pickles, soups (not the creamy kind), and mushrooms.

The FOOD 4 LIFE
Traffic Signal

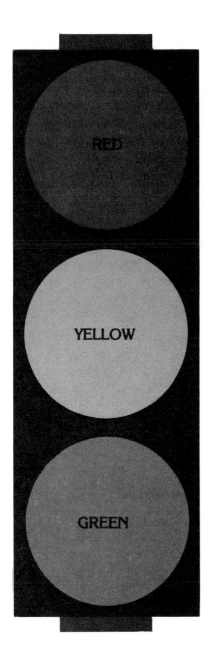

STOP eating things like cake, candy, red meats, ice cream, peanut butter, and cookies.

Eat with CAUTION when you see things like eggs, fruits, peas, potatoes, cereals, and milk.

GO ahead and eat things like asparagus, lettuce, broccoli, carrots, pickles, vegetable juice, and tomatoes.

RICHARD'S FOUR-STEP EASY EATING PLAN

1. Learn to recognize red, yellow, and green foods.
2. Learn the difference between real hunger and pretend hunger. (Real hunger is when your stomach growls and aches for some food. Pretend hunger is any other time you just feel bored and want something to do. It's during these times of pretend hunger that you're most likely to eat food your body can't use. And what happens when food is unnecessary? Right, it turns into fat. When you feel pretend hunger, do something else like reading a book, exercising, or going outside and enjoying the beautiful day. Better yet, talk to somebody about your feelings.)
3. Eat only when you feel real hunger.
4. Eating *too much* of a good thing can be just as bad as eating the wrong thing, so stop eating before you feel full.

CHAPTER 6

You Can Do It!
I Know You Can!

So this is our book. Our message is simple and direct and as hard as hell to execute: You can exercise your body and practice good nutrition NO MATTER WHAT. We want to spread this message to every man, woman, and child who thinks that a physical challenge puts you on life's sidelines.

Tim Green and Cheryl Abalu are the instructors for the very first Reach Foundation exercise class for the handicap-able, held at Orthopaedic Hospital, Los Angeles. When they announced that I was writing this book to help spread our message, the people in the class decided to write and tell me what the Reach program has meant to their lives.

My dream is that no child will ever again sit on a bench during P.E. class. The people whose letters I share with you now have that same hope, but *they* tell it better than anyone ever could:

Dear Richard,

I would like to take this opportunity to thank you from the bottom of my heart for making it possible for me to attend your Reach Foundation exercise classes.

Tim and Cheryl are fabulous. They both work on a one-to-one basis with us and the special attention we get from them is very helpful. Tim throws that dynamic energy that he possesses to me and I am motivated even though I am feeling the burn in my body.

I am really improving. I can now touch my knees with my elbows while sitting in my wheelchair, something I could not do at the beginning. I am still far from my goal in being able to make my left arm reach up and stay there, but Tim says we'll work on it.

Your sponsoring this program for us is a blessing. God will help you in every way because you are so unselfish.

Gratefully yours,
Cecelia

To the Reach Foundation:

What the Reach exercising class had done for me is that it has made me a better person by making me exercise. I thought all the exercise I could do was to be in a therapeutic pool doing non-weight-bearing exercises. Little did I know that I could exercise in my chair or on a mat.

It's easier to exercise in a group than by yourself. To see other people exercising in wheelchairs makes me want to do it too.

Since I've started exercising, it has helped me use my stomach muscles for something other than eating. My body feels great now, although in the beginning I had some muscle soreness. Now my muscles are getting in tone. The exercise helps me work out my frustration and makes me sweat, although I have to take it easy with any hip exercises because I don't have hip joints on either side. I must limit the movement in my hips or it causes internal bleeding in the hip area. The stretching exercises and movement of the head and neck are wonderful.

The exercises are excellent for me; they have given me a more pleasant attitude and given me a better outlook on life. Thanks to Tim and Cheryl; their encouragement is really wonderful.

> Thank you,
> Juan

Dear Richard,

I have benefited from the program not only for exercise, but getting out and being with people. Before I used to stay in my house and I did not go anyplace. Now I am learning to do things that I thought I had forgotten.

I had a mini stroke on my cerebellum and it left me unable to read or write. (As you can guess, a friend is copying my words.) I am learning to write my name again and also remembering my phone number. This program has allowed me access to exercise and as a result, I can even clap my hands. I can also stretch now as I could not before. I am able to walk better now too.

> Sincerely yours,
> Martha

Hi,

Just a little note to let you know that I enjoy the exercise sessions very, very much.
Since I've been coming to the classes, I feel much better and more relaxed.
Keep up the good work!

> Thanks again,
> Mavis

Dear Richard,

This class has not only opened my eyes to a new field of physical fitness, but it's also opened the eyes of my able-bodied friends. Suddenly, the people who share my life are interested in what types of exercises I am doing and how I am doing them.

Since the class, many other new and exciting things have developed in my life. I believe one of the most important things that has taken place is the fact that I have stopped smoking. I believe that if it wasn't for this class, I would not have stopped. I decided to get into better shape, and smoking while I was exercising seemed to be defeating the purpose! Next I've discovered stomach muscles! Being able to do fifty or more sit-ups without cramping is a big improvement for me. I actually feel good when I wake up in the morning and feel sore stomach muscles. It's a wonderful feeling because I know I've worked hard the night before and the class is actually working for me! Another exciting development was a real live muscle cramp in my left leg. Now that might not sound so exciting to anyone else, but believe me—if you've never experienced a leg cramp before, it's wonderful when you do. That means that things are starting to work for the <u>first</u> time.

Finally, my mental attitude has grown and developed since I've joined this class. I've realized how eating right and exercising regularly can change how you feel not only physically, but mentally as well. I find myself looking at the ingredients on packages to see how much sugar, salt, etc., they have in them. I've also started to lose the weight I've carried with me for years.

I want to thank everyone who has been involved with this class, but I especially want to thank God for blessing us with two very special people, our instructors, Tim and Cheryl.

Love,
Melody

Dear Richard,

I have been attending your exercise program since it began.

As an adult, I have had a weight problem and since I began to exercise, my weight has decreased. Whereas before I exercised, I was continually gaining weight.

As far as my muscles are concerned, I am now able to bend over in my wheelchair and come back up without using my hands. The stretching has helped me due to the fact that I am being stretched in the opposite directions of the way I sit in my wheelchair.

Sylvia

[One of the instructors added this note to the bottom of the letter: "P.S. As I've told Sylvia, her mental attitude has greatly improved!"]

Dear Richard,

I am 28 years old and have had cerebral palsy since birth. My left side is weak and the exercise class is helping me. I enjoy coming to your classes and I feel good after I exercise. I feel that I am getting stronger.

I enjoy all of the new friends that I have met at this class (especially my instructor).

Thank you,
Cindy

Dear Richard,

In two weeks I have exercised with no brace. I have progressed a great deal. With time and patience, I will accomplish more.

I am overjoyed because I have improved. I had a stroke on my right side. Thank you for Tim and Cheryl. I still have to straighten out my fingers on my right hand.

Yours truly,
Susie

Dear Sir,

Just to let you know that the exercise class has helped me quite a lot. Especially my neck, shoulder and elbow. This class has really helped the swelling in my elbows and knees.

Thank you,
Gloria

Dear Richard,

To evaluate this class in words is beyond words. Coming to this class has motivated me into doing so many things. I found strength and joy working out with so many joyful people. I think Tim is doing a wonderful job and I hope he can continue doing it.

Martha

Dear Richard,

This class has given me a better idea of how far I can exercise my physical abilities. The instructor is really sweet and full of energy. He makes you feel like doing the exercises! So here's to you, Tim!

Cindy

Dear Richard,

I look forward to going to your exercise program twice a week because I do not do them here at home. I enjoy doing them in a group.

I had a stroke in 1982 and it partially paralyzed my right side, so therefore I am in need of exercising. I appreciate your program because it helps me a great deal. I enjoy the individual attention that I get from Tim and Cheryl. Thank you.

Sincerely yours,
Lillian

Dear Richard,

Your exercise program is very good for me because I get out of my home and do something worthwhile. The exercises are fun and I really try very hard to do the different types of exercises. I have cerebral palsy so some of the exercises are difficult, but I am in there trying!

Thank you for this opportunity to help myself, and I will continue to come to your classes.

Sincerely yours,
Fernando

To the Reach Foundation,

I have been attending your exercise classes since February 1985. Since then I have gained great progress in my body, weight and mind. This is the most excellent program that's ever been established.

My thanks to Richard Simmons for his sponsorship and most of all to my instructors Tim and Cheryl for their dedication and time.

Again, thank you all and more power to you.

Sincerely,
George

[The instructor added this note: "George is now independent in his wheelchair. He can get to the floor from his chair, and back again without assistance. He never thought he could do that."]

To whom it may concern:

The "Reach" program has helped me in these ways:

1. <u>Strength</u>: Because of the exercise, my body has become stronger and I have more endurance. The exercise has strengthened the muscles around my loose hip prostheses, giving me better control when I walk.
2. <u>Flexibility</u>: Due to the stretching exercises, I now have more movement in my hips and shoulders, the joints that were stiff, "stuck" or "frozen" due to lack of movement.
3. <u>Sense of Well-Being</u>: The exercise seems to turn negativity into positive energy. Since I have started exercising, I am feeling happier with myself. Being a shy person, I am gaining more courage and more determination to do the best I can. Also, the exercise releases stored-up tension blocks. Since I have been coming to the "Reach" program, I have made less trips to the chiropractor for the release of tension knots. I especially enjoy the exercising with music. The music helps to take my mind off of the discomfort or difficulty I might be experiencing with certain movements. Tim has an excellent way of motivating us, and knows how to use humor to make that which seems impossible become reality.
4. <u>Discipline</u>: It is good for me to have a regular and definite time set for exercising. The "Reach" program forces me to make a real effort to do something positive with my body. I am now becoming aware of my body again, moving out of a stagnant state. After many hip surgeries it's easy to give up and just let your body go. It feels good to "try" again!

The "Reach" program is the best thing that has happened to me for a long time.

Thank you,
Nancy

APPENDIX

The Reach Foundation has an advisory committee including physicians, physical therapists, psychologists, nurses, nutritionists, occupational therapists, and social workers. These professionals work hard every day helping people discover how to meet physical challenges. And so before beginning this project, I asked them about any medical factors which might conflict with your program of general exercise and for any exercise and nutrition tips that other people had learned. We all agreed that the best thing to do was to contact as many experts as we could and "just ask them." And so we requested information from over 100 agencies, hospitals, and rehabilitation centers that were considered leaders in the field of exercise and nutrition for people with physical challenges. The responses we received make up the following appendix. It contains a lot of information that's never been put together in one place, and I know you're gonna learn a lot from it. (And not just about your own challenge!) But if your specific physical challenge is not included here, show the book to your doctor and ask just where YOUR exercise and nutrition program should fit in!

As you read this appendix, remember that these are only *general* principles and precautions. Because you are a *unique* person, your individual exercise and nutrition program must be planned with input from your own doctor or therapist.

AGING

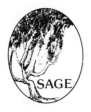

Consultant:

Helen G. Ansley, B.A.
—Member of the National Institute of
Health's SAGE project, 1974–75

OrthopædicHospital

Consultant:

Mark Wellisch, M.D.
Orthopaedic Hospital
—Clinical Instructor in Medicine
University of Southern California
School of Medicine
Los Angeles, CA

Definition

Isn't this terrible?!! There are actually people out there who see the aging process as a disability. Here you are at the peak of your sensitivity and maturation— a person with experience and wisdom— and you may look at your body as a worn-out old phonograph: too squeaky and stiff to give it another whirl. That's ridiculous! And my friend Helen G. Ansley, a consultant on aging and one of the original members of the Senior Actualization and Growth Exploration (SAGE) research project, thinks so, too. Helen is eighty-four years young and still running ahead of most people.

Some of the concerns older people have about movement and exercise come from the complications of weak muscles, stiff joints (often arthritic), heart problems, or high blood pressure. Each of these conditions can be complicated by poor muscle tone, inadequate nutrition, shallow breathing practices, and fat,

fat, and more fat. When you're a silver citizen, the easiest way to get fat is to slow down your activity and to keep up your old eating habits.

Common Psychological or Behavioral Barriers to Exercise

Lots of times, you may feel isolated and depressed. Sometimes, on the worst days, this loneliness can make you wonder why you should bother to do anything, let alone exercise. If you feel this way, you're wrong. You're not alone in your feelings, it's true, but you are definitely WRONG. A little bit of exercise each day can actually make you less depressed. And the reasons for that are physical as well as psychological. When you exercise you increase the amount of oxygen pumping around in your body, and that includes those sites in your brain that control your moods and emotions. More oxygen means that you feel better, you think better, and you *are* better. Besides increasing your oxygen flow, regular exercise also increases levels of adrenaline and noradrenaline. These are the "get-up-and-go" hormones that Mother Nature was so nice to give us all. Lots of researchers have proved that for several hours after exercise the presence of these hormones can give you feelings of increased energy, alertness, and self-confidence. And so you accomplish something pretty important when you exercise. The work you put into the activity can give you sincere feelings of reward and achievement. And if you exercise in a group, working, laughing, and sharing with others help even more.

Specific Nutritional Concerns

If you live alone, it's easy to skip meals and veggies, isn't it? Be honest. Sometimes you have a pot of tea and a bag of cookies for dinner, right? Well, you shouldn't do that! Please, pay particular attention to Chapter Four and the FOOD 4 LIFE program.

Specific Precautions for a Program of General Exercise

Watch out for dizziness and losing your balance. You can begin an exercise by holding on to a chair or another person. (That last one is definitely more fun!) Dizziness can also occur if you execute an exercise with a little too much "vigor" (the medical professionals call it postural hypotension). If you feel dizzy, take a couple of deep breaths and sit down. In fact, most of the exercises in Chapter Three can be done in a sitting position!

Stretch every muscle and bend every joint EVERY day, but don't forget to do it gently!

When I asked Ms. Ansley if she had any advice for those of us looking forward to healthy, happy silver years, she reminded me of a quote from Henry Ford: "'Whether you think you can, or think you can't, you're right!'" Then she added, "And have fun!"

ALZHEIMER'S DISEASE

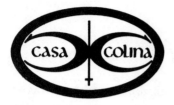

Consultants:

Bill La Franchi
—Director
   Adult Day Health Center

Jodi Brandenberger
—Alzheimer Program Coordinator
   Casa Colina Hospital for Rehabilitative
     Medicine
   Pomona, CA

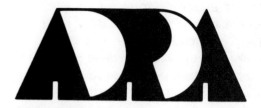

Consultant:

Stephanie Multer Goor
—Executive Director
   Alzheimer's Disease and Related
     Disorders Association, Inc.
   Los Angeles, CA

Definition

In the past, we incorrectly believed that everybody lost some intellectual functioning as he or she got older. The common phrase for this was "senility." But as scientists learned more about the brain they discovered that, first, not everybody gets senile and, second, senility is actually several different diseases. Since it affects 2 to 3 percent of the general population, Alzheimer's disease is the most common cause of severe intellectual impairment in older adults.

No one yet knows what causes this disease, but it does seem to follow a pattern. In the early stages, a person with Alzheimer's will function like everybody else. Soon, he or she will need to be reminded of simple things like the names of people, the date, or the correct time. Gradually, this "forgetfulness" turns into severe memory loss, confusion, irritability, restlessness, and agitation in personality. The disease is progressive (the symptoms continue to worsen), and it affects every person individually. Occasionally, change comes fast, but for most people intellectual impairment slowly increases over a period of years. In the later stages of the disease, the individual with Alzheimer's loses all ability to function independently.

Specific Medical Considerations

A person's medical and physical conditions depend entirely on the stage of Alzheimer's and his or her general health before the onset of the disease. Some people with Alzheimer's also have an assortment of so-called geriatric diseases that may require specific precautions, but if you're otherwise healthy, you should exercise every day. It won't reverse the effects of Alzheimer's disease, but it can relieve some of the tensions you're feeling. And some doctors believe that motor skills are retained longer if regularly exercised.

Common Psychological or Behavioral Barriers to Exercise

In the early stages of this disease, you may want more than anything to continue functioning as you always have. And so keeping your body in top form, and planning and carrying out a regular exercise program can make you feel better.

As the disease progresses, more and more daily activities will be supervised by a "caregiver" (often a family member). Now the major barrier to exercise can be the attitude of this second person. As intellectual functioning declines, it's harder for those around the person with Alzheimer's disease to keep up the pattern and routine of exercise. If you are the caregiver, it's gonna be necessary for you to schedule exercise, begin the activity, and frequently repeat even the simplest instructions. Try to keep to the same pattern each day so that the person with Alzheimer's is not faced with any confusion or new learning situations. In more complicated step-by-step exercises, it's best to be a model and exercise with the person you are helping. And you cannot always expect someone with this disease to understand verbal commands such as "Raise your right leg." Instead, you will need to demonstrate the action or give cues like touching the part of the body to be moved. Most important, recognize that the person you are helping to exercise *physically* needs this activity to maintain joint strength, muscle tone, and overall flexibility.

In the later stages of the disease, it will be especially necessary to coordinate an exercise program with a doctor or physical therapist. An intense exercise program may not be available as the person begins to lose a sense of body awareness.

Specific Nutritional Concerns

Currently, there are no nutritional restrictions for a person with Alzheimer's, but as the disease progresses, choosing and preparing a well-balanced diet become very confusing. In later stages, there will even be difficulty in using utensils or chewing large pieces of food.

Many people with this disease experience a period of time during which they always feel hungry and will literally eat any food they can reach. Later, they may lose any interest in food and need to be fed by the caregiver.

Specific Precautions for a Program of General Exercise

If you are a caregiver for someone with Alzheimer's, it's very important that you keep any exercise program well within the individual's tolerance level. Keep exercise sessions short (less than thirty minutes), and constantly be on the lookout for signs of fatigue. Dizziness and falls are very real possibilities for people in the middle or late stages of the disease. If this is true, exercising in a chair will still allow the person to increase cardiovascular circulation and to exercise the long muscles of his or her arms and legs. The best forms of exercise for the person with Alzheimer's are those containing familiar movements. Learning is difficult and eventually impossible, so use exercises that may have been learned in school or the military. These might include toe touching, jumping jacks, or running in place. Walking is another excellent exercise, particularly if you follow the same path and point out things along the way.

Warning Signs of Physical Overextension

The warning signs of overextension (especially for the person taking psychotropic medications to control anxiety and delusional thinking) are shortness of breath, generalized weakness, a change in color (flushed or pale), rapid heart rate, and clammy skin or profuse sweating. If any of these symptoms occur, stop exercising immediately. If this should happen, a person with Alzheimer's may become confused and/or frightened, and so it's essential that the caregiver stay until the symptoms stop. Give reassuring comments such as "I will stay with you," or "You will be okay."

If you are helping care for a person with Alzheimer's disease, you are a very important person. Establishing and maintaining an exercise routine *will* help make every day the best it can be. You must have patience and enthusiasm, and still keep your realistic perspective. But while you're doing all of that, please, don't forget to take a little time for yourself.

AMPUTATION
(including congenital limb malformation)

OrthopædicHospital

Consultants:

Timothy B. Staats, M.A., C.P.
—Adjunct Assistant Professor
  Director
  Prosthetics-Orthotics Education
    Program

Yoshio Setoguchi, M.D.
—Medical Director
  Child Amputee Prosthetics Project
  UCLA School of Medicine
  Los Angeles, CA

Consultant:

David W. Edelstein, M.D.
—Director
  Amputation Clinic
  Orthopaedic Hospital
  Los Angeles, CA

Definition

Amputation is the surgical removal of a diseased or irreparably damaged or non-functional limb. Currently, there are over 1.5 million amputees in America, and every year an additional 40,000 to 50,000 amputations are performed. The most common reasons for limb amputation are vascular disease (caused by conditions such as arteriosclerosis or diabetes mellitus), trauma that interrupts the blood supply (such as automobile or industrial accidents), burns or severe frostbite, and infections that may or may not be life threatening. While any of these factors may occur at any age, malignant tumors, accidents, and congenital malformations are the most common reasons for amputations during childhood. Eighty-five percent of all amputations occur in the lower extremities.

Amputation of an arm or a leg creates a residual or remnant limb (commonly called a stump). Improved surgical methods and the technology responsible for new prosthetic devices (artificial limbs) mean that once the stump has healed, almost any amputee can and should exercise.

Specific Medical Considerations

When amputation has occurred because of a disease, that disease is more of a consideration than in the actual amputation. For example, in the case of arteriosclerosis, a person may also have signs and symptoms of coronary-artery insufficiency or claudication pain (cramping) in remaining limbs. And people with amputations from a malignancy may need to plan their exercise programs around chemotherapy and/or radiation treatments. If this is true for you, be sure to plan your exercise program with the help of your physician.

In the case of congenital malformation, however, the child rarely has other medical conditions that would interfere at all with regular exercise.

All of this is to say that you are an individual, and once the stump created by the amputation has sufficiently healed, your program of exercise will also be individual.

Common Psychological or Behavioral Barriers to Exercise

Each of the experts I spoke with pointed to "body image" as the greatest barrier to any physical activity. The fitting of a prosthesis can go a long way in restoring your self-esteem, but real confidence comes only when you can resume and master activities you did before the amputation. And the best way to do this is to get the rest of your body in top physical condition!

Tim Staats, director of UCLA's Prosthetics-Orthotics Education Program, told me that timing is also important: "The immediate shock of the loss of a limb can be followed by relief, knowing that one has survived a serious illness. Later, some people become depressed when their expectations of 'Six Million Dollar Man' replacements are not reality. When he or she finally comes to grips with reality and adapts his or her life to a new set of rules—then there is no upper limit to performance. Amputees have sky dived, SCUBA dived, played baseball, football, and tennis, and even run across the United States!"

Dr. Yoshio Setoguchi, medical director of the Child Amputee Prosthetics Project, UCLA School of Medicine, finds that the greatest stress in this situation is often that felt by family members. Parents are anxious about how a child with a congenital limb malformation will grow and develop. In these cases, he feels that the entire family must be counseled regarding the stress the child will experience as he or she tries to compete with peers; stress due to stares, hurtful comments, and teasing from other children; and the challenges of normal social, recreational, and athletic events.

When it comes to the amputee child growing up, Dr. Setoguchi said, "It should be strongly emphasized that the majority of limb deficient or amputee children do not need *special* exercise programs. In fact, special programs should be discouraged! The more these children are allowed to participate in 'normal' activities, the better."

Specific Nutritional Concerns

It's important to consider the underlying cause of the amputation. For example, if you have arteriosclerosis, you must follow the diet prescribed by your physician.

If you are an adult with an amputation and have no other health problems, you must keep your weight at a constant level so that your prosthesis will fit. It may seem minor to anybody else, but a few pounds gained or lost can mean a new artificial limb.

In Chapter Four, FOOD 4 LIFE, we use insurance scales and formulas to help you determine your ideal weight. But none of the regular statistics works if you have a missing limb. Even so, there is a neat calculation you can use to modify these numbers. The following tells you the body-weight percentages of each limb. Multiply the appropriate percentage by your ideal weight (see chart on page 125) and subtract that number from the weight listed on the chart.

Body Part	Percentage of Total Body Weight
Arm	6.5
Upper Arm	3.5
Lower Arm	2.2
Hand	.84
Lower Leg	7.1
Total Leg	18.7

Specific Precautions for a Program of General Exercise

Dr. Setoguchi cautions the parents of a child with an amputation to evaluate carefully exercise programs, instructors, and sports equipment before the child begins any activity. Safety is a real concern, particularly since growing children must have the fit of a prosthesis adjusted regularly. He reminds you that an ill-fitting prosthesis and improper exercise instruction can cause injury. The best advice is that you teach your child to recognize signs of fatigue and stress so that he or she can become self-regulatory.

Hygiene of the amputation site is especially important for both adults and children. A stump sock or liner that's soiled with perspiration can cause skin irritation and discomfort, and thus keep you from exercising. Tim Staats suggests that you cover your stump with polyethylene sheeting (plain old Saran Wrap) and clean your prosthesis with alcohol to control perspiration buildup.

If you wear your prosthesis during an activity, proper fit and an appropriate construction are your best precaution.

Some prosthetic devices are designed only for walking, not heavy activity. As Tim says, "Nothing is impossible for an amputee to do physically, however, the cost of replacing an artificial limb which gets broken due to inappropriate or unexpectedly heavy use can be prevented." So save yourself some aggravation and money by planning ahead.

If you don't wear the prosthesis during exercise, protect your stump from bruises and scratches by wrapping it with an Ace bandage.

One final precaution—for the safety of others: Pad your prosthesis. An artificial limb is made of hard plastic and metal—and when somebody runs into it, he can get hurt!

Warning Signs of Physical Overextension

Dr. David Edelstein, director of Orthopaedic Hospital's Amputation Center, said, "The only general warning sign I can think of is stump pain due to skin irritation. Otherwise, each person should consider any primary medical problem that may have been the reason for amputation. If for example, a person has arteriosclerosis, he should stop exercising and contact a physician if he experiences: chest pain, rapid heart rate, dizziness, nausea, or any of the other warning signs his physician has already given him.

"Every amputee is an individual and so exercise programs must be individualized. But unless the person is medically unable to exercise (as in extreme senility or end stage heart and lung problems) he or she should be encouraged to follow a regular and vigorous exercise program."

Although some sports require special equipment and prosthetic adaptations, amputees can participate in ALL sports activities. If you feel you're ready to extend beyond a program of general, daily exercise, you might want to contact some of the people helping to organize competitive activities for the person with an amputation:

Jack East
American Amputee Foundation
710 S. Gaines St.
Little Rock, AR 72201

Kirk M. Bauer
National Handicapped
  Sports and Recreation Association
Suite 201
1200 15th St. N.W.
Washington, DC 20005

Dick Bryant
U.S. Amputee Athletic Association
Rt.#2, County Line Rd.
Fairview, TN 37062

National Amputation Foundation
12-45 150th St.
Whitestone, NY 11357

Superkids (a newsletter for families of
  children who wear prostheses)
60 Clyde Street
Newton, MA 02160

AMYOTROPIC LATERAL SCLEROSIS

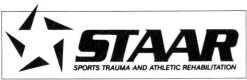
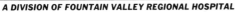

A DIVISION OF FOUNTAIN VALLEY REGIONAL HOSPITAL

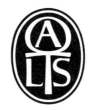

Consultant:

Alan M. Strizak, M.D.
—Medical Director
 STAAR Institute
 Fountain Valley
  Community Hospital
Fountain Valley, CA

Consultant:

Jean O'Shea
—Operations Manager
 The Amyotropic Lateral Sclerosis
  Association
Sherman Oaks, CA

Definition

Amyotropic lateral sclerosis (ALS) is a group of progressive, degenerative diseases of the spinal cord and brain. Nobody yet knows its cause, but it is one of the more common neurological disorders affecting adults. Known more popularly as Lou Gehrig's disease, ALS strikes individuals between the ages of forty and seventy (men are affected twice as frequently as women). More than 250,000 Americans now living will develop the disease, and scientists suspect that millions more may possess the neurological predisposition for ALS. For most people, ALS quickly progresses to paralysis and death. But the ALS Association reports that many of these deaths result from the treatable complications of the disease. But for 20 percent of the people with ALS, the disease may plateau for many years or even permanently stop for some unknown reason.

While organizations such as the ALS Association and the Muscular Dystrophy Association continue trying to find the cause and, thus, cure of the disease, most patients and physicians concentrate on coping with its effects. For many people, these can include progressive muscular weakness and an involuntary lack of emotional control (inappropriate laughing and/or crying are very common). Generally, ALS will not affect your senses (touch, taste, sight, smell, hearing), nor will it alter your intellect.

If you have ALS, you're probably very concerned about losing your independence. You want to keep your lifestyle and daily activities as long as possible. Exercise and good nutrition can help you do this.

Specific Precautions for a Program of General Exercise

Not only will exercise make you feel better, but it will also help prevent joint stiffness and muscle spasms and cramping. Your only precaution is that you carefully listen to your own body and avoid exercises that would be fatiguing. You and your doctor will probably plan your exercise program around the stretching and range of motion exercises seen in Chapter Three. Start out slowly, and gradually add more repetitions as you feel like it. Follow the pattern of warm-up, short exercise period, rest period, short exercise period, and cool-down.

Warning Signs of Physical Overextension

Stop exercising if you notice any of the following: extreme fatigue, a rapid or irregular heartrate, shortness of breath, dizziness, or nausea.

ARTHRITIS

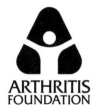

ARTHRITIS FOUNDATION

Consultants:

Diane Ross-Simon, M.P.H.
—Vice President
  Medical Education Program

Mary Rosenberg, R.P.T.
—Physical Therapist
  Arthritis Foundation
  Southern California Chapter
  Los Angeles, CA

Definition

Actually, there are more than 100 diseases lumped together under the term "arthritis." But they'll have some common denominators: pain (sometimes constant, but usually intermittent), stiffness, and usually some inflammation in one or more joints.

If you have arthritis, you are joined by almost 40,000,000 other Americans, young and old. And you have this disease for life. Nobody knows the cure, and, except for a few kinds of infectious and inherited arthritis, nobody knows the real causes. While some kinds of arthritis can be brought on by trauma to the joints (such as a sports injury or an auto accident), other types are thought to be triggered by a virus.

The most common forms of the disease are rheumatoid arthritis and osteoarthritis. Of these two, rheumatoid arthritis is usually considered the most serious since it can begin with a chronic inflam-mation in the tissues surrounding a joint and then (if untreated) can cause disease in the lungs, skin, blood vessels, muscles, heart, and even the eyes. By contrast, osteoarthritis has little or no inflammation and usually does not affect the whole body. It is this second and most common form of arthritis that we usually associate with advanced age. Experts at the Arthritis Foundation tell me that almost every person over the age of sixty has some form of osteoarthritis, and so it's no surprise that some doctors call it the "wear and tear" disease.

My grandmother had arthritis, and I think one of the things that made the disease so difficult for her was what therapists call the "on-again, off-again" syndrome. Some days she would seem to be perfectly healthy, and other days she would be unable to move her hands and legs. It was easy for other people to think she was just complaining to get attention. I know this must have been very frustrating for her as she would "push on" in pain and accepted the disease as simply a part of getting older.

Specific Medical Considerations

Most people can use medication (primarily aspirin) and moderate exercise to maintain the health of their arthritic joints. But if your arthritic joints have lost normal motion (either because of the disease or because of long-term inactivity), then you may not be able to exercise them. (Now, don't get all excited. This doesn't mean you get to watch *General Hospital* while everybody else is at exercise class. All of the rest of you needs exercise! Arthritic fingers will not interfere with leg lifts.) So it's very important for you to check with your doctor to see if moderate exercise would either strengthen or harm your diseased joints.

Common Psychological or Behavioral Barriers to Exercise

Mary Rosenberg, a registered physical therapist and volunteer with the Arthritis Foundation, tells me that people with arthritis often do not exercise because of their feelings about pain. It's easy to think that if you're in pain and if you *hold real, real still* then the pain will go away. That's not always true. In fact, long-term inactivity can actually *increase* both the pain and the damage started by the disease.

Finally, chronic pain can do terrible things to your spirit and to your soul. If you have arthritis, your greatest battle can be in keeping that positive, enthusiastic personality that is the *real* you.

Specific Nutritional Concerns

Because so many people suffer the chronic pain of arthritis and because there are no known cures, there are lots of shady characters out there making a fast buck on home remedies, special diets, and super vitamins. The only thing that ever gets healthier in these deals is the guy's bank account.

(Actually, gout is the only form of arthritis that may improve when you avoid foods such as kidneys, liver, sweetbreads, sardines, anchovies, meat extracts, and alcohol.)

Good nutrition and a normal weight *are* important in the control of arthritis since extra fat puts unnecessary stress on arthritic joints. I mean, for heaven's sake, why make it worse than it is?!

Specific Precautions for a Program of General Exercise

The key point is to *think* about your own body. Think about which joints are diseased, and plan your program accordingly. If you have arthritis of the spine or in any joints in your legs, then you should avoid running, jumping, or any other "pounding" type of exercise that will put stress on your diseased joints.

By the same logic, don't put pressure on your hands (such as with push-ups) if your hands are arthritic. Avoid bending your head and avoid sit-ups if the arthritis is in your neck. Do not practice sit-ups, bending at the waist, or pulling down toward your toes if you have arthritis in your lower back. And do not kneel on knees affected with arthritis.

So what can you do?!? Aerobic exercises, bending and flexing muscles, stretching, and slowly moving a joint through its range of motion (ROM) are the best exercises for arthritic joints. An example of a simple ROM exercise would be to hold your hands palm down in front of you and slowly rotate your wrists as far as they will comfortably go. First in a clockwise rotation, then in a counter-clockwise rotation.

Warning Signs of Physical Overextension

If you experience extreme fatigue or if you begin to feel increased pain that lasts for more than one or two hours, contact your doctor for specific instructions.

Mary gives you this final checklist for beginning your exercise program:

—— Before exercise, warm up the arthritic joints with a heating pad, hot moist towels, or a warm shower.

—— Exercise with very low repetitions (two to five of each exercise).

—— Pace your exercise program as you would pace your daily activities.

—— Rest before you get tired, and

—— Break your daily exercise program into two or three short sessions instead of trying to do it all at once.

ASTHMA

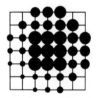

NATIONAL JEWISH CENTER FOR IMMUNOLOGY AND RESPIRATORY MEDICINE

Consultants:

Ann G. Guthrie
—Director of Rehabilitation

Michael LaMothe, R.P.T.
—Physical Therapist

Ronald L. Davis, T.R.S.
—Recreation Therapist

Lisa Norling, T.R.S.
—Recreation Therapist
    National Jewish Center for
        Immunology and Respiratory Medicine
    Denver, CO

Los Angeles Chapter

ASTHMA & ALLERGY FOUNDATION OF AMERICA

5410 Wilshire Boulevard, Suite 1008 • Los Angeles, California 90036 • (213) 937-7859

Consultants:

Scott E. McCreary
—Executive Director

Roger M. Katz, M.D.
—Director
    Los Angeles Chapter
    Asthma & Allergy Foundation of America
    Los Angeles, CA

Definition

Asthma is a complex disease that from time to time causes the obstruction of a person's respiratory system. All kinds of metaphors have been used to describe the sensation: "Breathing through a straw" or "hungry for air" seem to be the most common. But in acute asthma, there is a feeling of extreme panic as you struggle to catch your breath. An estimated 9,000,000 Americans experience asthmatic symptoms that can be caused by such factors as allergens (things you're allergic to, like certain foods, pollen, chemicals, animal hair, etc.), climatic conditions, emotions, viral infections, and *exercise*. This last factor is gonna give us some interesting things to talk about. Eighty percent of people with asthma have a condition referred to as "exercise-induced bronchospasm" (EIB for short). Sometimes an intensive aerobic exercise session of only five minutes can cause chest tightness, shortness of breath, wheezing, coughing, stomach- and headaches, and dry throat.

So why's asthma in a book about exercise? Betcha thought you were excused, right? WRONG.

I have asthma. So does Jacklyn Joyner, 1984 Olympic silver medalist in the heptathalon. And so do hundreds of thousands of athletes and physically active individuals.

How? We control asthmatic episodes with medication and/or self-monitoring. There are medications, for example, that if taken shortly before rigorous exercise can "block" the narrowing of airways. (The most common include atropine sulfate and isoproterenol, but your physician will be the one to fill you in on the details.)

Self-monitoring means self-control of stress, environment, and diet. For example, if your asthma is triggered by an allergy, you must learn to identify which substances cause the reaction, where they are, and how to *avoid* them. Lots of times this means not eating your favorite foods or finding a new home for a beloved pet.

Exercise-induced asthma is complicated, but it, too, can be modified or controlled. Dr. Roger Katz, a director with the Asthma & Allergy Foundation of America, says that EIB can occur after only five minutes of very strenuous exercise and usually within five to fifteen minutes after you've stopped. Symptoms can last from two minutes to two hours, and they usually go away by themselves. (Although you may need to inhale an aerosol medication if the episode is severe.) And so you can control EIB by taking medication before exercise and by working at shorter and less intense exercise periods. Another interesting aspect of EIB is that you can help prevent it if you will exercise again within one hour of an EIB reaction. Now I understand why my grade-school history teacher told us that Teddy Roosevelt had asthma but he got better when he went out west and climbed mountains. *Controlled* exercise helps you control EIB!

Common Psychological or Behavioral Barriers to Exercise

Listen, nobody wants to exercise if he thinks it's going to make him choke to death! An asthmatic reaction can leave you with feelings of panic and helplessness.

But *not* exercising and *not* getting involved in the physical activities of your peers can also be bad. Dr. Katz told me that for kids, this lack of participation very often leads to low self-esteem. Lisa Norling, a recreation therapist with the National Jewish Center for Immunology and Respiratory Medicine, agreed. "When asthma limits a person's physical activities, he or she often becomes lonely or depressed. People with asthma can become isolated from peers and have difficulty forming relationships."

Having asthma is not easy, but you CANNOT pamper yourself. With proper medication, self-monitoring, and self-control, you can and SHOULD exercise EVERY day.

A Note to Parents

We can't talk about asthma and behavior without talking about temper tantrums. Almost every therapist I talked to mentioned the fact that many children with asthma use the threat (consciously or subconsciously) of an asthmatic episode to manipulate family members. What can I say? Asthma is in your lungs, not your head. You are HURTING, not helping, your child if you let him use his asthma to get his own way. Mention it the next time you see the doctor or therapist—it could start a very important conversation.

Specific Precautions for a Program of General Exercise

Michael LaMothe, a physical therapist with National Jewish in Denver, suggested that you follow these guidelines:

—Do not bounce when doing stretching exercises.

—Be sure to do a warm-up session before exercise and a cool-down session after exercise.

—Use your prescribed medications BEFORE exercising.

Warning Signs of Physical Overextension

Even with all your precautions, asthmatic reactions can occur during exercise. Stop exercising if you notice extreme shortness of breath, severe wheezing or tightness in your chest, rapid pulse rate, or total exhaustion.

Michael had this final bit of advice for you: "Feeling a little frightened about exercise is normal. But if you remember to take your medications properly and regularly, you'll do fine. Most of all, relax and enjoy yourself!"

BACK PAIN

OrthopædicHospital

Consultants:

Mark Wellisch, M.D.
—Attending Physician
  Orthopaedic Hospital
—Clinical Instructor of Medicine
  University of Southern California
    School of Medicine
  Encino, CA

Lorraine Snow, Ph.D.
—Clinical Psychologist
  Pain Control Center
  Orthopaedic Hospital
  Los Angeles, CA

Definition

Back pain can be caused by lots of different things—congenital conditions, disease, or injury—but for the millions of people affected by this condition the key element is always the same: PAIN. In fact, much of your life is spent trying to forget, prevent, or stop what is often long-term (or chronic) pain.

Common Psychological or Behavioral Barriers to Exercise

Because back pain can be constant and draining, it usually causes two extremely difficult emotional states: anxiety and depression. Both can keep you from exercising.

The anxiety can come when you're afraid to move because you think you might hurt your back again. But inactivity just makes things worse! If you don't exercise your muscles, they become weak, and when they become weak you stand a greater chance of hurting yourself when you do something simple like bending over to smell a flower or reaching down to pick up the cat. It's a vicious circle. If you add obesity to the formula (something that usually happens when you stop moving and keep on eating), then you've got even bigger troubles.

Dr. Lorraine Snow, a psychologist who helps a lot of people with chronic back pain, tells me that you can get pretty discouraged when you don't even feel like getting out of bed, let alone exercising. In fact, Dr. Snow says depression and back pain are so interconnected that it's hard to tell which is the chicken and which is the egg.

By now *I'm* anxious and depressed just talking about all of this anxiety and depression! Thank goodness there's something we can both do about it!! (You get three guesses and it rhymes with *schmexercise.*)

As Dr. Snow says, "When done properly, exercise can actually protect some-one from injury. It's just a matter of get-ting up and doing it, even when you don't feel like it!"

No doubt about it. Exercise:

strengthens your muscles and thus helps prevent further injury to your back,

makes you feel proud of yourself and your body, and

makes you feel too good to be anx-ious and depressed.

Specific Precautions for a Program of General Exercise

Before you start fulfilling all these prom-ises of good times, you've got to have a plan.

Dr. Mark Wellisch of Orthopaedic Hos-pital in Los Angeles put it this way. "Exercise is of paramount importance to recovery. In fact, almost no disabled back patient recovers without a regular exercise program. But if not carefully tailored to individual problems, limita-tions and state of recovery, exercise can make the problem worse."

So ask your physician to approve any of the exercises you select and to give you specific instructions. Once you get started, keep these general rules in mind:

—If you feel a sharp pain—STOP!
—Avoid exercises that arch your back.
—When lifting, always use your legs, not your back.
—Avoid sudden, twisting, or jerky motions.
—Start with sitting exercises and grad-ually build up to those in which you stand.

Finally, if you haven't exercised for a while, you're bound to feel some sore-ness and discomfort. Don't give up—your body's just telling you that it's about time you got it moving again. Go a little slower the next day if that helps, but just keep going! Later, as the soreness goes away, you can add more exercises. The important point is that you keep a con-stant pace and that you keep telling yourself, "This is for me—and I'm gonna feel great!"

Warning Signs of Physical Overextension

IF IT HURTS, STOP! (Did I say that al-ready? Never mind. It's worth repeating.)

CANCER

Consultant:

Susan J. Mellette, M.D.
—Professor of Medical Oncology
   and Rehabilitation Medicine
—Director
   Cancer Rehabilitation Program
   Medical College of Virginia
   Richmond, VA

Consultant:

Carolyn A. Russell, L.C.S.W.
—Oncology Social Worker
   Los Angeles, CA

Definition

Cancer is a term used to describe over 100 different diseases. It is characterized by the uncontrolled growth and spread of abnormal cells. Normal cells reproduce in an orderly manner and grow for a purpose, such as to replace worn-out tissues or to repair injuries, but cancer cells grow for no apparent reason. They multiply uncontrollably, destroying normal cells and often spreading to other parts of the body.

Specific Medical Considerations

Since cancer can occur anywhere in the body, the medical considerations are determined by the place where the cancer has been found and the method used to treat it.

Frequently, the cancer is removed by surgery. If this is the case, then your exercise program would focus on the particular area affected. Very specific exercise programs will be prescribed by your physician after certain types of surgery. These include procedures involving the head and neck, the breast, or the limbs.

If radiation therapy has been used to treat the cancer, the specific treatment site may be inflamed like a sunburn. Depending upon the site and the individual, radiation can also cause diarrhea, a difficulty in swallowing, mouth soreness, and a decline in the sense of taste. Many people also experience a general feeling of fatigue and physical weakness when undergoing radiation therapy, but these symptoms usually disappear when treatment is completed.

Chemotherapy (the use of medications) is a treatment used to destroy those cancer cells that are not within easy reach of surgery or radiation, or to destroy cancer cells that remain after these two procedures. Sometimes chemotherapy can produce reactions such as nausea, vomiting, diarrhea, anemia, and a lowered resistance to infection. If you are receiving chemotherapy and experiencing these symptoms, they can usually be controlled by your physician.

Even people who have cancer that has spread to other parts of the body can benefit from a general exercise program. Such a program may enable them to maintain mobility and functions.

Common Psychological or Behavioral Barriers to Exercise

The greatest psychological impact of cancer is almost always universal: fear. This can be a fear of pain, a fear of the unknown course of the disease, and ultimately a fear of death. Each person expresses this fear differently, but common reactions are anger, anxiety, depression, loss of appetite, and withdrawal. This makes stress a very crucial part of the cancer experience. And as we all know, exercise can help reduce stress!

Maybe you're afraid that exercise will worsen your condition, make you weak, or cause pain. But the opposite should be true! And if you set realistic and appropriate goals, exercise will not only maintain and build muscle strength, it can also lift your spirits and give you a positive self-image.

Specific Nutritional Concerns

Most people who have completed treatment for cancer will not have specific nutritional concerns. If the cancer was located in the gastrointestinal tract (esophagus, stomach, intestines, or colon), you may have some dietary precautions such as avoiding highly seasoned, spicy, or hard to digest foods. If this is true for you, check with your physician or a trained dietitian who has had experience with cancer patients.

Dr. Susan Mellette, a cancer specialist, and Carolyn Russell, an oncology social worker, both told me that nutritional concerns are more of a factor if you are currently receiving radiation or chemotherapy. For example, if you're experiencing side effects of these treatments, you may not be able to eat very much at one time or keep it down when you do eat. It's best for you to eat small amounts several times a day and to eat foods that are high in both calories and nutritional value. The National Cancer Institute in Bethesda, Maryland, and the American Cancer Society both have developed books that provide specific nutritional information and recipes designed for cancer patients receiving radiation and/or chemotherapy. (You can get free copies of these books from your local American Cancer Society office.)

They both gave me a word of caution here: There are numerous clinics and individuals who promote diets, vitamins, nutritional plans, and counseling that they claim will cure cancer. NONE of these has ever proven to be a cure, and many are considered to be fakes or frauds! The people peddling these plans take your money and give you only false hope. More important, they may cause you to turn away from legitimate treatments that could eliminate, arrest, or reduce your cancer. So before talking to anyone who advertises such a "magical diet," check with your local American Cancer Society office for information.

Specific Precautions for a Program of General Exercise

Anyone who has had recent surgery should get specific exercise instructions from his or her physician. For example, if you have had abdominal surgery, you may need to postpone exercises like sit-ups, but these same exercises could be very beneficial at a later date. Most important, don't overdo it. There's no reason to do too much too fast.

Some specific examples could include:

—If your cancer has been surgically removed, you may be able to return gradually to your former physical condition, maintain it, and build more muscle strength.

—Some types of chemotherapy may result in temporary muscle weakness, so if you are receiving such chemotherapy, you may want to discuss this with your doctor.

—If the cancer has spread to your bones, they may become very brittle and you may need to avoid jogging, aerobics, or jumping exercises.

Warning Signs of Physical Overextension

Most of all, exercise should not be painful. Stop exercising if you experience joint or bone pain or if you feel dizzy, sick, or light-headed.

Carolyn had these final thoughts for you: "Exercising is a very individual thing. The sooner you start after treatment for cancer, the easier it will be in the long run to maintain your muscle tone. When you begin an exercise program, you are doing something positive for yourself! You are expressing faith in your future."

CEREBRAL PALSY

Orthopædic*Hospital*

Consultant:

Karen J. Gilman, M.S.W.
—Legislation and Advocacy Coordinator
  United Cerebral Palsy
    Spastic Children's Foundation
  Van Nuys, CA

Consultant:

Wilfred Krom, M.D.
—Clinical Professor of Orthopedics
  University of Southern California
    School of Medicine
—President, Medical Staff
  Orthopaedic Hospital
  Los Angeles, CA

Definition

Cerebral palsy is a group of conditions involving nerve and motor dysfunction and is caused by damage to the developing brain. This damage may occur before birth or it can be the result of a childhood injury or illness. Everyone with cerebral palsy responds in a different way, but basically it means that you have difficulty controlling the actions of your body. You think, reason, and feel just like everybody else, but involuntary and jerking body movements, muscle spasms and seizures, and problems with speech, hearing, or vision can interfere. In other words, your body doesn't easily respond to the mental commands you give it.

Specific Medical Considerations

Muscle tightness and limits to body movement depend very much upon the type of cerebral palsy and upon the location and severity of any brain damage.

However, thousands of people with cerebral palsy (and other neuromuscular disorders such as muscular dystrophy, multiple sclerosis, and arthogryposis) have decided that a problem with movement would not prohibit them from leading busy, active lives. And the United Cerebral Palsy Association has developed a fantastic program of competitive athletics under the direction of The National Association of Sports for Cerebral Palsy. Local teams train and compete in state, regional, and national events in sports such as archery, horseback riding, power lifting, table tennis, wheelchair and ambulant soccer, bocci, bowling, rifle shooting, and track and field events. All participation is based upon individual abilities and a complex series of skill categories. For example, someone with quadriplegic involvement may throw a four-pound shot put while an athlete with minimal involvement would throw an eight-pound shot put.

Common Psychological or Behavioral Barriers to Exercise

When I asked Dr. Wilfred Krom, about any special psychological problems you may experience because of CP, he said, "Most persons with cerebral palsy do not have any more psychological involvement than do persons in the general population."

Specific Precautions for a Program of General Exercise

As with other neuromuscular disorders, you need to check with your physician before beginning your exercise plan. Some people with the spastic form of cerebral palsy, for example, should not include stretching in their exercise programs. Medication, extent of any reoccuring seizures, joint condition, and the health of your cardiovascular system also must be considered before you begin.

Warning Signs of Physical Overextension

Dr. Krom says that you should stop exercising if you notice breathlessness, an irregular or excessive heartrate, overheating, dehydration, or pain in an individual joint.

Dr. Krom also adds these words of encouragement, "Get involved—set your goal (such as arm strengthening, better wheelchair control, etc.)—and work diligently at it."

CHRONIC OBSTRUCTIVE PULMONARY DISEASE
(Chronic Bronchitis and/or Emphysema)

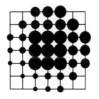

NATIONAL JEWISH CENTER
FOR IMMUNOLOGY
AND RESPIRATORY MEDICINE

Consultants:

Ann G. Guthrie, R.P.T., M.S.A.
—Director of Rehabilitation

Michael LaMothe, R.P.T.
—Physical Therapist

Lisa Norling, T.R.S.
—Recreation Therapist

Ronald L. Davis, T.R.S.
—Recreation Therapist
National Jewish Center for
Immunology and Respiratory
Medicine
Denver, CO

Definition

Chronic obstructive pulmonary disease (COPD) is a term that includes the diseases of chronic bronchitis and emphysema. Chronic bronchitis is defined as a chronic or recurrent productive cough that can be caused and/or irritated by factors such as influenza, bacterial infection, asthma, pollution, and smoking. Emphysema is a disease in which the tiny air sacs in the lungs are slowly but permanently destroyed, causing the creation of larger (and less efficient) air sacs and eventual inflammation of your lungs. The result of this tissue damage is that your lungs cannot supply the rest of your body with oxygen, and that in turn leads to complications throughout your system. Both diseases follow a slow, progressive process. The first symptoms may be dismissed as a cold, but they recur often and become more severe as the lung tissue becomes more damaged and susceptible to infection. Breathing becomes very hard work.

But none of this excludes exercise. In fact, experts such as those with the National Jewish Center for Immunology and Respiratory Medicine have determined that if you continue to exercise and eat well, you will be in better health and function more effectively than will someone who just sits around "taking it easy." The trick is to begin a program that gradually increases your tolerance to exercise and movement.

Common Psychological or Behavioral Barriers to Exercise

This disease gives you the feeling that you have no control over your life, and that in turn has a way of lowering your self-esteem. You may have to change drastically your lifestyle and profession, and this leads to additional tensions and pressures. You've got to work hard to overcome feelings of depression and anxiety. This is the point at which a program of gradual and regular exercise can give you more control over your body and your ability to move.

Specific Nutritional Concerns

Diet is very important if you have COPD. In the early stages, you've got to watch calories very carefully because carrying around extra fat only adds to the difficulty you have breathing. But as the disease progresses, you may find that eating is the last thing you want to do. Now diet control will probably mean maintaining proper calorie and protein levels so that you won't lose muscle mass after all the fat's burned off. If you are at this point, your physician will prescribe a specific dietary plan.

Specific Precautions for a Program of General Exercise

Ronald L. Davis, a therapist with National Jewish, told me that there are several precautions you should follow before beginning your exercise program:

—Have a cardiac screening *before* exercising to detect any possible heart disease or heart failure.

—Have a physical assessment for structural (neuromuscular/skeletal) problems *before* exercise.

—Remember that you should *gradually* increase your tolerance for exercise and you should follow the pattern of warming up, exercising, and cooling down.

—Avoid any vigorous, rapid, and sustained exercise. Rest often and pace yourself.

—Avoid jumping and any movement that requires you to tilt your head downward or hold your arms overhead. Concentrate instead on more static exercises and those you can do while sitting.

—Be sure to use any medication or oxygen that your doctor may have prescribed.

—Never hold your breath while exercising.

Warning Signs of Physical Overextension

Stop exercising and consult your doctor for further instructions if you notice any rapid and distressful breathing, tightness in your chest, wheezing, high pulse rate, dizziness, loss of balance, nausea, or skin discoloration.

Remember to begin slowly and gradually add an exercise as you feel more capable. Exercises in the sitting position are the best for you if you have COPD, but swimming, graduated stair climbing, walking, and static stretching exercises can also allow arm and leg movements without extraordinary stress.

Ronald Davis said it this way: "The management of COPD can be a frustrating and burdensome task. Beginning a program of physical fitness may seem to present an impossible challenge if the exercise involved cannot be made accessible and rewarding. But gainful change can be achieved if you will embrace a total approach including proper exercise modifications, breathing retraining and family support. For almost every level of this illness, a strategy of rehabilitation and exercise can be the best prescription."

CYSTIC FIBROSIS

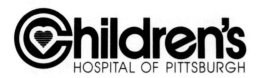

Consultant:

David M. Orenstein, M.D.
—Member of the Professional Education
  Committee
—Foundation Consultant in Exercise and
    Cystic Fibrosis
  Cystic Fibrosis Foundation
  Rockville, MD
—Director
  Pulmonology Division
—Director
  Cystic Fibrosis Center
  Children's Hospital of Pittsburgh
  Pittsburgh, PA

Consultant:

Robert J. Beall, Ph.D.
—Executive Vice President for
    Medical Affairs
  Cystic Fibrosis Foundation
  Rockville, MD

Definition

Cystic fibrosis (CF) is the most common life-threatening genetic disease of children within the white population. Twenty years ago, the stereotypic image of a child with CF would include adjectives like "scrawny," "sickly," and "sedentary." But our knowledge and maintenance of this disease have so advanced that a more accurate image may be of a teenage boy or girl who regularly jogs or swims.

The exact biochemical details of CF are still unknown, but the major clinical result of the disease is an accumulation of abnormally thick mucus that can clog the lungs and pancreas. When the pancreas is so clogged, the body cannot completely absorb nutrients from food. This in turn leads to problems with growth and development. The more serious complication, however, occurs in the lungs. When mucus prevents the free movement of air, lung tissue becomes progressively scarred and infected.

Many children with CF, their family members, and physicians feel very strongly that exercise improves the conditions of the disease. They believe that activity will make you feel better, and as a result you will be able to do more. Lots of scientists have been studying this effect, and while exercise may not change pulmonary function, it can increase fitness and tolerance to more exercise, and (along with physical therapy) help you cough up and expel mucus from your lungs.

Common Psychological or Behavioral Barriers to Exercise

Dr. David Orenstein, Children's Hospital of Pittsburgh, said: "There are *no direct* psychological or behavioral problems from cystic fibrosis. In fact, it's remarkable how well most patients with CF cope with what can be a difficult physical situation. However, the diagnosis of an inherited, chronic, incurable disease may affect family functioning. As this disease becomes progressive, some patients and families need support to cope with its impact."

Specific Nutritional Concerns

Cystic fibrosis patients lose considerably more salt in their sweat than do people without the disorder. (This fact has received much publicity as new parents are told to advise a physician if they "taste" salt when kissing their children.) As a result, a child with CF should be given free access to the saltshaker.

Specific Precautions for a Program of General Exercise

The specific way in which CF has affected your lungs will determine the kinds of exercises that will be best for you. And so before beginning to exercise, plan your program with your physician.

In order to prevent severe salt loss, avoid prolonged exercise (more than several hours) during hot weather and be sure to consume adequate amounts of liquid and salt. (Salt tablets are not necessary and are probably not helpful.)

Warning Signs of Physical Overextension

The warning signs for someone with cystic fibrosis are exactly the same as those for anyone else. These would include shortness of breath, rapid pulse, dizziness, nausea, and extreme fatigue.

Dr. Orenstein concluded, "For the large majority of patients, including those with severe pulmonary problems, exercise can be extremely beneficial and enjoyable. Keeping with the theme of this book—it's probably true that almost *no one* with cystic fibrosis *can't* exercise."

DIABETES

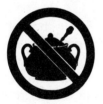

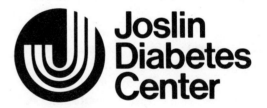

Consultants:

Barbara Toohey
—Director
June Biermann
—Cofounder
  Sugarfree Center Inc. for diabetics
  Van Nuys, CA

Consultant:

Marilynn Gay Montgomery
—Member, American Diabetes
    Association
  Cofacilitator ADA Support Groups
  Pasadena, CA

Consultant:

Charles A. Graham, M.D.,
  Joslin Diabetes Center
  Boston, MA

Consultant:

Evelyn J. Basile-Gay, M.D., F.A.A.P.
—Staff Physician
  New Mexico State University
  University Park, NM

Definition

Diabetes is a metabolic disease affecting 12,000,000 Americans. The cause of diabetes is still unknown, but we do recognize two types of the disease: Type I, insulin dependent diabetes, which primarily affects children and young adults; and Type II, non-insulin dependent diabetes, which usually affects adults.

Diabetes occurs because of a malfunction in the body's supply of insulin. As your body absorbs nutrients, insulin is the hormone (produced by the pancreas) that keeps blood sugar within normal limits. It works something like a catalyst or a key opening the door to body tissues so that sugar (or energy) can enter and thus provide nourishment. If insulin is not present, is present in insufficient amounts, or cannot be absorbed, the door stays locked; the sugar stays outside the tissue and it isn't nourished. When this happens, the blood sugar level rises and a person has diabetes.

An uncontrolled blood sugar level can eventually cause complications such as diabetic retinopathy (resulting in blindness) and kidney failure. Often, injuries of the extremities fail to heal, and this in turn can lead to gangrene and/or amputation. People with out-of-control diabetes also have a higher incidence of high blood pressure and associated cardiovascular complications (such as stroke, heart attack, and arteriosclerosis).

Even though this sounds terrible, people with diabetes can and do live "normal" lives. They do this by controlling their blood sugar levels with diet, insulin or oral hypoglycemic medications, and exercise! Even the three-sided logo of the

American Diabetes Association emphasizes these three vital elements. And of the three, exercise is probably the most neglected—and the most feared and misunderstood.

Specific Nutritional Concerns

If you have diabetes, you're already on a diet prescribed by your physician. You'll probably find that the FOOD 4 LIFE food plan (Chapter Four) is similar to what you're eating now—but you should STICK TO YOUR PRESCRIBED DIET.

Specific Precautions for a Program of General Exercise

In the past, doctors debated whether exercise helped or caused problems in diabetes management. Now it's universally understood that if you follow certain precautions exercise is very beneficial to blood sugar normalization. Marilynn Gay Montgomery of the American Diabetes Association told me that if you have diabetes the most common problem you may have during or following exercise is a rapid drop in your blood sugar level. This often results in a condition called hypoglycemia (or low blood sugar reaction), and it's something you want to avoid. The symptoms of hypoglycemia (also called insulin reaction) are sweating, a pounding heart, trembling, dizziness, disorientation, and disrupted thought patterns. If left untreated after such a reaction, you *could* become unconscious and even die.

The fear of having one of these hypoglycemic reactions may have kept you from exercising on a regular basis. It shouldn't! While the risk of reaction is present, you can learn to anticipate and control it. Moreover, the cardiovascular benefits of regular exercise are too important for you to ignore. The best way to relieve any fear is to discuss your specific insulin therapy and your specific exercise needs with your doctor. If you have diabetes, you're not gonna be able to come home from work one day and decide to run a four-minute mile before dinner. You've got to plan your exercise program, diet, and insulin control program well in advance. Decide to do it today—talk to your doctor today—but exercise only after you've made diet and insulin adjustments.

After you and your doctor have designed your exercise program, you can learn to monitor your blood sugar level with a simple device. Before, during, and after exercise, you can obtain a small drop of blood from your fingertip (there's even a special little tool for this) and put the drop on a reagent strip. The strip can be visually read for color changes and interpreted by a small, calculator-size colorimeter. The result? An instant blood sugar reading. You can use this instant information to avoid any insulin reaction.

Once you've learned how to use the monitoring device, your specific precautions include the following:

—Carry emergency glucose! Dextrosols, BD glucose tablets, Glutose, Dextrogel, Lifesavers, or even sugar cubes will do the trick.

—Wear comfortable, broken-in shoes plus socks. Do not get blisters! Blisters for you can mean real problems later. People with diabetes sometimes don't heal as rapidly as other people, and so it's best simply to avoid injuries in the first place. If you have neuropathy or poor sensation or circulation in your feet, check them after every exercise session to make sure they have come through uninjured.

—If you have diabetic retinopathy (an eye problem characterized by leaky blood vessels), check with your doctor before doing any exercise that involves bouncing, jumping, jogging, jiggling, dancing, or placing your head lower than your heart.

—Always eat prescribed meals and snacks in the proper amount and at the proper time before and after exercise.

—Ask your doctor to tell you when your insulin "peaks" and try not to exercise during these periods. This will lessen the chance of hypoglycemic reaction.

—Exercise with a friend who understands diabetes.

—Always wear diabetic emergency identification jewelry. An "I Have Dia-betes" card in your wallet isn't going to do you any good if you go jogging in your shorts and T-shirt.

—If you're really concerned about a rapid drop in blood sugar, take the blood sugar testing kit with you when you exercise. Then you can periodically monitor yourself and avoid any unnecessary fear about hypoglycemia.

Warning Signs of Physical Overextension

Stop exercising if you feel any of the symptoms of hypoglycemia: sweating, trembling, rapid heartrate, dizziness, disorientation, and/or disrupted thought patterns. Check your blood sugar or urine sugar and contact your doctor if you even suspect an insulin reaction.

DOWN'S SYNDROME

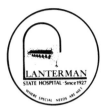

Consultants:

Lorenda M. Vergara, M.D.
—Acting Medical Director
—And the staff of Lanterman State
  Hospital and Developmental Center
  Pomona, CA

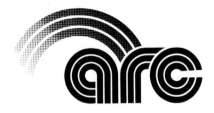

Consultants:

Dixie Henrikson
—Executive Director

Mary Schallert
—Assistant Director
  Activities for Retarded Children
  North Hollywood, CA

Definition

The hereditary units that tell our bodies how to develop are called genes. Hundreds of genes are linked together to form larger units, and these are called chromosomes. Every cell in the bodies of most people contains forty-six chromosomes. Those individuals with forty-seven chromosomes are said to have Down's syndrome. We don't fully understand what causes this difference, but the extra chromosome disturbs the orderly development of the body and brain, and so people with Down's syndrome share specific physical and mental characteristics. As with everybody else, there is a great range and variety among people with Down's syndrome, but the most common of these characteristics include some reduction in body and head size; a broad, short neck; a prominent abdomen; short fingers and toes; mild malformations of the creases and furrows in fingers, palms, and toes; a generalized muscular hypotonia (often leading to slow and uncoordinated movements); and mental retardation. The degree of mental retardation varies considerably in each individual, but the average mental age is eight years. People with Down's syndrome also exhibit specific facial characteristics. These include an upward and outward slope of the eyes, a flattened forehead, a high and narrow palate, full cheeks (often with a reddish tint), enlarged nostrils, smaller than normal ears (sometimes contributing to hearing loss), dental malformations, and generally soft and fine hair. Because of other facial malformations (specifically, a relatively narrow nasopharynx, enlarged tonsils and adenoids, and the protrusion of an enlarged tongue) people with Down's syndrome habitually hold their mouths open.

Specific Medical Considerations

People with Down's syndrome often have higher incidences of congenital heart disease (and this in turn can also lead to delays in gross motor development), hip dislocation, and acute lymphoblastic leukemia. They are unusually susceptible to infections, especially respiratory infection. Generalized abnormalities of the musculoskeletal system often result in joints that are lax and hyperextensible (which means "loose" and can result in a slower and less coordinated walk). Up to 10 percent of all persons with Down's syndrome also experience a condition known's as Atlantoaxial dislocation. This is a misalignment of two cervical vertebrae in the neck, and it can play an important factor in exercise. (We'll talk about it again later.) Finally, there seems to be a higher incidence of Alzheimer's disease in older adults with Down's syndrome.

Common Psychological or Behavioral Barriers to Exercise

A great deal of research has been devoted to what have been called the characteristic personality and behavioral traits of people with Down's syndrome. Nobody likes to be placed in a sterotypic mold, and every doctor or therapist will be quick to tell you that there are considerable individual differences in every person with Down's syndrome. But Dr. Lorenda M. Vergara, medical director of Lanterman State Hospital and Developmental Center, described some of the behavioral and personality traits often seen in people with this condition: "People with Down's syndrome have considerable power to imitate and a strong sense of the ridiculous. This last point is indicated by their humorous remarks and the laughter with which they hail accidental falls. They exhibit great obstinacy and can be guided only by consummate

tact—no amount of coercion seems to induce them to do what they have made up their minds not to do.

"Thus people with Down's syndrome cannot be *pushed* and they have a difficulty in taking criticism. They must be coaxed and led and learn best from *life modeling.*

"Much as others do, people with Down's syndrome thrive on being complimented on their efforts, and respond better to low key enthusiasm."

These behavioral characteristics are particularly important if you are helping a person with Down's syndrome plan and execute a program of regular exercise and nutrition. As is often the case with anyone having mental retardation, a person with Down's syndrome is slow to learn new ideas and patterns of behavior. But be patient and consistent! Once learned, these patterns are also very slow to *unlearn.* So if you help teach someone with Down's syndrome how to eat properly and exercise regularly, he or she will probably carry these habits throughout life.

Specific Nutritional Concerns

Many people with Down's syndrome become obese. Some doctors feel this is metabolic and that people with Down's syndrome should consume even fewer calories if they are to maintain an ideal weight. Nevertheless, if you're the parent of an overweight child with Down's syndrome, it's primarily *your* fault. You buy the food and you put it on the table. Read Chapter Four and learn about the FOOD 4 LIFE program. Begin teaching your child which foods he may or may not eat. Make sure that you don't bring high-calorie, low-value foods into your home! And if you child attends a specialized school or sheltered workshop, check out the kinds of food on the premises. If you find high-calorie junk, raise a fuss with the administrator until things change!

There is evidence that specific mineral and vitamin supplements will improve muscle tone and hypotonia, and because of Down's syndrome patients' tendency toward dry skin and sparse hair growth, Vitamin A has often been prescribed. This is an individual matter and should be checked out by your doctor.

Specific Precautions for a Program of General Exercise

Because so many factors associated with Down's syndrome can influence the ability to move, begin an exercise program only after a complete physical examination. One important element of that exam is whether or not your child as Atlantoaxial dislocation (a displacement of neck vertebrae). Stretching or flexing the neck of a person with this condition could lead to severe and permanent spinal cord injury. So if you have any doubt, avoid any exercises that include a hyperextension (stretching) of the muscles of the head and neck. Your doctor will use a neurological examination and X rays to diagnose an Atlantoaxial dislocation, but the symptoms of the condition are a deterioration in ambulatory skills, changes in bowel or bladder function, changes in neck posturing, neck pain or a limitation in neck movement, and a weakness of an extremity.

Some other suggestions mentioned by Dr. Vergara:

—Begin slowly and gradually add exercises as stamina increases.

—Encourage group activity.

—Include antigravity exercise (like swimming).

—Avoid exercises that involve hyperextension (stretching) of major joints (this can cause dislocation).

—Avoid exercises that require heavy lifting or performance on a narrow base of support (like walking a balance beam).

—If osteoporosis is present, avoid any jolting type of exercise (especially along the vertical axis of the body).

—Avoid rotary action along the vertical axis of the spine, even if the person is sitting.

—Keep a person with Down's syndrome from holding his or her breath when moving.

—Carefully monitor any person with cardiac problems (your doctor can give you specific instructions).

And finally, Dr. Vergara told me that you must have additional patience when teaching any exercise with excessive eye-hand coordination and any exercise with multiple sequencing (step-by-step) instructions.

Warning Signs of Physical Overextension

Unless a person with Down's syndrome has severe mental retardation, he or she can be taught to recognize many of the following warning signs. However, if you are a parent or the supervisor of the exercise program, stop exercising if you notice reactive hyperemia (congestion or a red skin color), chest pain, profuse perspiration, hot flashes and dizzy spells, headache, sustained tachycardia or bradycardia, shortness of breath, hyperventilation, blue lips (cyanosis), discolored extremities, pain and swelling of a joint secondary to dislocation, back pain, sustained tremors or seizures, abdominal pain, esophageal spasm, a lack of self-control (incontinence), continuous coughing, or confusion.

There are some activities that are particularly beneficial for anyone with Down's syndrome (or other forms of mental retardation). Dr. Vergara included some of these for your exercise plan:

- When possible, stress sequencing exercises, which coordinate action of two hands and/or legs (*i.e.,* jumping jacks, four-limb crawl, two-hand pulling, or throwing with two hands).
- controlled kicking with bent knees
- jumping in place with bent knees
- working against resistance (going up and down stairs, riding a stationary bicycle, using a rowing machine)
- swimming
- rolling up hill

If your child has Down's syndrome, you already know that you've got to provide extra amounts of patience and planning for any activity. But please don't overlook daily exercise and good nutrition! You're trying so hard to help your child reach his or her fullest potential. Obesity and weak or flabby muscles only give him an extra "handicap" he doesn't need.

The best way for you to start is by being a model and a guide. Today—this very minute—start your own program of exercise and proper eating. Your child will follow your example and you both will be winners.

EPILEPSY

OrthopædicHospital

Consultant:

Shirley Whiteman, M.D., F.A.A.P.
—Pediatric Coordinator
    Spina Bifida or Birth Defect Team
    Orthopaedic Hospital
    Los Angeles, CA
—Pediatric Instructor
    University of Southern California
        School of Medicine
    Los Angeles, CA

Consultant:

Gerald I. Sugarman, M.D., F.A.A.P.
—Pediatric Neurologist and Genetic
    Consultant
    Glendale, CA

Definition

Epilepsy is not a disease, but a set of symptoms that come about when there is a specific disorder of a person's central nervous system. Brain cells of the person with epilepsy create abnormal electrical discharges, and these in turn cause the person to temporarily lose control of some body functions. The lack of control (seizures) can include muscle spasms, mental confusion, a loss of consciousness, and/or uncontrolled body movements. Seizures can be mild or severe, but they usually last for only a few minutes. In the past, we were all told to put a stick or a chalkboard eraser in the mouth of someone having a seizure. That advice caused lots of unnecessary injuries. If you are present when someone with epilepsy has a seizure, you should: stay calm!; remove any hazards like utensils, furniture, etc.; gently turn the person's head so as to clear and protect the airway; leave the person where he is unless he's in a clearly dangerous place (like a street); let the seizure run its course (don't call a doctor unless it lasts for more than ten minutes). When the seizure ends, the person may be slightly disoriented or embarrassed—so most of all, be reassuring and thoughtful.

Before we knew anything about epilepsy, people who experienced these reactions were denied employment, socially outcast, and feared. Fortunately, epilepsy can (in most cases) be controlled with medication. And when he's not having a seizure, a person with epilepsy is just like everybody else.

The cause of epilepsy has been linked to birth defects, severe head trauma (usually after a loss of consciousness), diseases, infections, poisons, tumors, or metabolic disorders (from poor nutrition). But nobody is exactly sure *why* such seemingly unrelated events could prompt an epileptic seizure.

Dr. Shirley Whiteman told me that if you have epilepsy you need exercise and good nutrition as much as anyone else. However, she stressed that you must avoid exercising to the point of fatigue. In fact, inducing first fatigue and then sleep is one way doctors have of prompting and observing an epileptic seizure.

Common Psychological or Behavioral Barriers to Exercise

Some people with epilepsy still allow the ignorance of others to keep them from being as active as they would like. And if you have epilepsy, you may believe the old stories about how you should be "disabled." But, particularly if your epilepsy is controlled with medication, you can do anything you want to do. There's absolutely no reason for you to sit in your room waiting for a seizure to occur. Besides, your body will get fat and flabby if you don't exercise every day. You can even still participate in outdoor activities like swimming, boating, mountain climbing—just take along a "buddy" who can help you if you have a seizure.

Yes, it's annoying to have to take regular medication and precautions, but thank God you have them to take! Quit using the fear of a future seizure as a reason to ignore today.

Specific Nutritional Concerns

For a few people, seizures may be caused by vitamin and/or mineral defi-ciencies. If this is true for you, your doctor will prescribe a special diet and supplements.

Otherwise, you need only follow the FOOD 4 LIFE food plan described in Chapter Four.

Finally, most doctors agree that you should avoid alcohol. It can really have negative effects when mixed with your medication.

Specific Precautions for a Program of General Exercise

As I stated earlier, you must avoid fatigue. Begin slowly and add exercises only as your stamina increases. Exercise a little less on those days you've been doing other physically demanding or tiring jobs, like cleaning out the basement or moving your office to another building. Unless you also have another physical challenge (in which case you should look it up in our appendix or talk to your doctor), you have the same general precautions as would anyone else: warm-up, exercise, and cool-down.

Warning Signs of Physical Overextension

Again, these signs are the same as for anyone else. Stop exercising if you notice extreme fatigue, rapid or irregular heart-rate, nausea, dizziness, breathlessness, or a severe pain in a joint or muscle.

FRIEDREICH'S ATAXIA

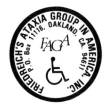

Consultant:

David A. Stumpf, M.D., Ph.D.
—Associate Professor of Pediatrics and
  Neurology
  Northwestern University
  Evanston, IL

Consultants:

Susan L. Perlman, M.D.
—Assistant Professor of Neurology and
  Anesthesiology

Becky Kern, R.P.T.

Nadia Simon, R.D.
  UCLA Special Inherited Neurologic
  Disease Center
  Los Angeles, CA

Definition

Friedreich's Ataxia is a hereditary condition that causes a lack of coordination both when moving your arms or legs and when speaking. In addition, it's often accompanied by heart disease, diabetes, and scoliosis (a curvature of the spine).

Dr. Susan Perlman of UCLA tells me that the person with Friedreich's Ataxia can often preserve muscle strength and slow the progression of the disorder with a regular program of exercise.

Specific Medical Considerations

Although strength can be preserved, the lack of coordination associated with Friedreich's Ataxia is progressive and may lead to the use of a wheelchair. But there are certainly many exercises that can be accomplished from a wheelchair. Most important, avoiding obesity and involving yourself in a regular program of exercise may actually slow the functional decline you experience.

Specific Precautions for a Program of General Exercise

Usually, exercises that increase your cardiovascular strength, breathing capacity, and spinal flexibility can be very helpful for you, but these kinds of aerobic exercises can be hard on joints and bones or (if your balance has been affected) increase the risk of falling. So check with your physician for a specific evaluation before you begin. Many people with Friedreich's Ataxia find that the same aerobic benefits can be obtained from using a modified exercise bicycle or by swimming.

If you are also diabetic, you should know that exercise can alter insulin requirements. Again, check with your physician.

In addition, a complication of Friedreich's Ataxia is often a slowing of reaction time, so avoid exercises that require quick movements. Slow, deliberate exercises like stretching and reaching would be much better.

Warning Signs of Physical Overextension

Dr. David Stumpf of Northwestern University suggests that you stop exercise if you notice any chest pain, palpitations, dizziness, or sudden shortness of breath.

The specialists of the UCLA Special Inherited Neurologic Disease Center have this last bit of advice for you: "Exercise may increase your fatigue, but brief rest periods will quickly restore your ability to stay active. Most importantly, try to exercise with others who have Friedreich's Ataxia. Group exercise is a wonderful way to keep your motivation high and to share thoughts and feelings."

HEAD TRAUMA/BRAIN INJURY

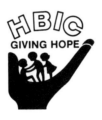

Consultant:

Thomas J. Ragain
—Rehabilitation Therapist
   Veterans Administration
      Medical Center
   Palo Alto, CA

Consultants:

Peggy Lasko, M.A.
—Director
   Fitness Clinic for the Physically
   Disabled

Peter M. Aufsesser, Ph.D.
—Coordinator of Adapted
      Physical Education
   San Diego State University
   San Diego, CA

Consultants:

Cleta J. Harder
—Executive Director

Peter S. Springall
—Sensorimotor Developmentalist
   Help for Brain Injured Children, Inc.
   La Habra, CA

Consultant:

Karl Knopf, Ed.D.
—Coordinator of Adaptive Physical
      Education
   Foothill College
   Los Altos Hills, CA

Definition

Every single one of us is vulnerable to neurological impairment caused by either injury or trauma (a blow to the head— most often in car accidents), vascular disease (such as a stroke, aneurysm, or heart disease), or a cerebral tumor. Head injury has been called the Silent Epidemic because with very little public awareness 50,000 new traumas occur every year. (And two-thirds of these people are under the age of thirty.)

When a normal healthy brain incurs such trauma or disease, the resulting disabilities vary according to the location and extent of the damage. For example, individuals with brain injuries could have problems with speech (the expression of words), language (understanding what is said to them), memory, or motor function. Thomas Ragain of the Veterans Administration is a man who works every day to help people overcome the effects of head trauma. He tells me there is a common misconception that brain injury always results in severe and permanent emotional, mental, and intellectual dysfunction. Rehabilitation (and this most certainly includes exercise and movement) can often work miracles.

The term "brain injury" is often used when discussing infants born with neurological dysfunction. For any number of physical or medical reasons, these babies will have developmental delays in areas such as language, fine and gross motor skills, and sensory competence. In the past, these children have been stamped with such misleading terms as "mentally retarded," "emotionally disturbed," and "slow learner." The terms are misleading because they all indicate a very low chance of improvement. People like Cleta Harder, executive director of Help for Brain Injured Children, Inc., works very hard to dispel these notions. She tells me that *every* child, regardless of the labels, should be given the chance to reach his or her highest learning potential. And her words have been put into action. Since 1967 she has been involved in the education of over 2,500 children and young adults with brain injury. She says of her teaching methods, "Every movement that a baby makes helps program its central nervous system. Therefore all activities and lessons are presented in the same sequential order that is seen in a developing infant without brain injury."

This same kind of "sequential training" is used with adults who have experienced brain injury. Old tasks affected by the injury are retaught, just as they had been during childhood.

Specific Medical Considerations

If you are a person with a brain injury, it is very likely that you may have been placed on a long-term anticonvulsant medication. Usually, this will not interfere with your normal activities, including exercise. But it is important that you check with your physician before initiating your exercise plan. A history of hypertension or any weakness or paralysis caused by your injury could mean that you shouldn't practice a specific movement.

Common Psychological or Behavioral Barriers to Exercise

Although there can be several physical/psychological effects on your behavior after a brain injury, Mr. Ragain feels that one of the most common is a decrease in your sense of self-worth. Lots of times he sees people who before the injury had taken health and physical abilities for granted. If you were such a person, it may be hard now to see beyond what you used to and now "can't" do. Here again, a successful exercise program can help you regain old strengths or build new ones.

To the person assisting someone with severe brain injury: As we've indicated, the term brain injury is very broad. Many times the injury will involve a condition known as aphasia. Aphasia can be temporary or long-term and is divided into two types: receptive aphasia (the inability to comprehend spoken language) and expressive aphasia (the inability to execute speech). If you are assisting a person with aphasia, consider the following guidelines from physical educators Peggy Lasko and Karl Knopf:

—Allow the person to make mistakes while speaking. Occasional corrections are okay, but if you correct too often he or she will not want to speak.

—Never interrupt a person with aphasia, and supply words only when help is requested.

—If a person with aphasia gives an unrelated response, casually restate the subject of the conversation.

—Build up confidence by emphasizing and praising the activities a person with aphasia can do.

—Don't take it for granted that a person with aphasia understands all that you have said. Occasionally repeat instructions.

—Keep material short, simple, and concrete.

—Use demonstration along with verbal instructions.

Specific Precautions for a Program of General Exercise

If your head injury is the result of a vascular accident (*i.e.,* a stroke), then it is especially important for you to monitor your blood pressure when exercising. (Your doctor can give you specific instructions on how this can be done.)

And if you have a history of hypertension, it is important that you avoid any exercise using strenuous weight lifting.

Sometimes a head injury can cause visual problems and if this is the case for you, be sure that you exercise in the "wide open spaces." Give yourself lots of room so that you won't crash into something when you do that first waist twist or hip flip.

And finally, if you have a shunt (a surgical apparatus that keeps cerebrospinal fluid in balance), you must avoid any exercise with an extreme neck movement. Examples of such exercises could be ones that involve abrupt hyperextension or flexion of the neck. (For example, gymnastic stunts such as forward and backward rolls, contact sports such as basketball or soccer, and diving.)

Warning Signs of Physical Overextension

Stop exercising if you notice any of the following: shortness of breath, severe headache, weakness and/or dizziness, an excessive heartrate, an abnormal blood pressure after exercise, residual fatigue (lasting for more than twenty-four hours), or insomnia.

Overall, it's best to approach exercise gradually. Avoid unrealistic or "instant" goals. It will take a while to regain the skills you had before the injury, but you *can* make progress. The best exercises for you will be those that involve:

- flexibility: stretching movements
- balance: balancing on your knees or on a balance beam (Be sure to use a spotter.)
- coordination: movements like jumping and hopping (Again, use a spotter.)
- cardiovascular strengthening: running in place or using a stationary bike

Peter Springall, sensorimotor developmentalist with Help for Brain Injured Children, Inc., also stressed the need for a consistent and intense program of developmental exercise. This means moving from simpler to more complex movements. And Peter suggested that you display a big, colorful chart of daily accomplishments and progress. It's a great motivator, 'cause everybody likes to see his name "up in lights."

HEARING IMPAIRMENT

*"...and the ears of the deaf
shall be opened."*

Consultant:

Victor Goodhill, M.D., F.A.C.S.
—Professor of Surgery
—Chairman of the Board
  Hope for Hearing Foundation
  UCLA Medical Center
  Los Angeles, CA

Consultant:

Lee Thomas Watrin
—Educator

Marilynn Gay Montgomery
—Educator
  Marlton School
  Los Angeles Unified School District
  Los Angeles, CA

Definition

Technically, a hearing impairment is any condition that interferes with a sound as it enters the ear and is interpreted by the brain. Such interference can be mechanical, as when the eardrum or the three small bones of the middle ear fail to function properly, or it can be neurological, as when transmissions are incorrectly received within the inner ear or the hearing center of the brain. There can be many different kinds of hearing loss, ranging from mild (even temporary) to profound deafness.

Common Psychological or Behavioral Barriers to Exercise

When I began the Reach Foundation, it never occurred to me that a person with a hearing loss would be included in our "target population." After all, I thought, your ears are a pretty small part of your body—the rest of you should be able to exercise just fine! But I was wrong. And as we began the pilot exercise classes for Reach, I was surprised to see many people with moderate to profound hearing loss join our classes. They had felt excluded from so-called mainstream exercise programs because of errors and omissions by the instructors.

Exercise instructors who could hear, myself included, assumed that people with hearing impairment could just watch us and "catch on." Not true. If you have a hearing impairment, you can get totally confused and lost in a mainstream exercise class. The instructor can turn his or her back and you lose the instructions. You don't hear the encouragements. And perhaps most important, you can't hear the music, judge the rhythm, and thus keep up with the group. You end up feeling like you're in an *I Love Lucy* rerun—always a couple of beats out of step.

If you *are* hearing impaired, be certain

to tell your instructor! A hearing loss is often called the hidden handicap because people can't *see* that you don't *hear*. When you tell people that you are "hard of hearing," "hearing impaired," or "partially deaf," it can be a good way to facilitate communication.

Next, you should ask your instructor where you should sit to see him best. Many people with hearing impairment "hear with their eyes," or read lips. So ask the instructor always to give instructions in the same place and always to face you.

But the best coping mechanism is to make friends! That way you can ask someone to repeat the directions and/or show you how to do the exercise.

As far as not hearing the music, there are several things you can do. First, you can watch the instructor of the class until you determine the cadence or rhythm of the exercise. Is it 1-2-3, or 1-2-3-4, or 1 and 2 and 3 and 4? Your classmates or the instructor can syncopate the rhythm for you by clapping it out. Or better yet, forget trying to keep the beat! Exercise to the beat of a different drummer! Just keep going! Don't stop! Do whatever is best for you.

But there are even more mechanical ways to solve the problem of rhythm. Lee Watrin, a teacher with the Marlton School in Los Angeles, told me that slight modifications in the physical structure of the exercise room can make mainstream exercise classes more accessible to people with hearing impairments. First, install speakers in or near the floor. This allows those with hearing impairments to actually *feel* the music and keep in step with the group. Second, place mirrors around the room so that people with hearing impairments can see the instructor from several angles

and thus pickup even slight body movements and visual cues.

If you wear hearing aids, you know what sometimes happens if you sweat profusely into those costly little guys, right? They short out or make *frying* or staticlike noises that can keep you from hearing at all. There are a couple of things you can do to prevent this disaster. First (if you're comfortable when you "wing it" with the instructions), take off your hearing aids while doing aerobic or "sweaty" exercise. If you take this course, be sure to tell the instructor that you're temporarily "off the air." (And for heaven's sake, be sure to put them in a safe place!)

Second, use a sweatband and keep a towel handy. If you frequently wipe off your brow and your hearing aids, you'll avoid a lot of problems.

Third, you can buy special products that dehumidify hearing aids. (Usually, the kit contains a plastic envelope and a special container of silica gel crystals. These crystals absorb moisture and dry out your hearing aids.) One note: Never, never try to dry your hearing aids by putting them in the oven and/or microwave! You'll melt and destroy the delicate instrumentation.

If you can't hear the instructor's encouragements, that can make it harder for you to stay motivated. But remember, the instructor *is* giving encouragements. Try to think positive thoughts. Look at the other people. Watch them move. You can tell it's hard for them, but they're not stopping—don't you stop, either! Play your own encouragement tape in your head and keep up the good work!

If you have a hearing impairment, *and* if you have no other physical challenge, there is no earthly reason why you should not be exercising *every* day. If you feel out of step in group programs, then develop one of your own. Ask some friends over (give the ones with full hearing some earplugs), and turn up the volume on your stereo. Feel the music and get moving!

Specific Precautions for a Program of General Exercise

Primarily, you need only follow the same precautions as any able-bodied person: Start slowly and gradually add exercises as your stamina builds. Look for any unusual signs such as extreme fatigue, dizziness, severe headache, rapid breathing, rapid heartrate, or any persistent pain in a muscle or joint.

A final precaution: If you exercise outside, jog, or walk, either wear your hearing aids or go with a friend. That way you will minimize the danger of being hit by a car or something.

HEART DISEASE

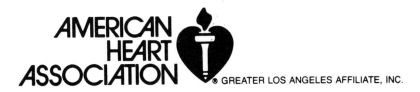

GREATER LOS ANGELES AFFILIATE, INC.

Consultant:

Michael J. Wong, M.D.
—President
  American Heart Association, Greater
    Los Angeles Affiliate, Inc.
  Los Angeles, CA

Definition

The term "heart disease" refers to dozens of separate diseases of the heart and blood vessels. Collectively, they account for over one half of all the deaths in America. And another 1.25 million people experience and survive heart attacks. Yet as grim as these statistics are, the rate of fatal heart disease has actually declined in the past twenty years. This is because we have learned what causes heart disease and how to prevent it.

There are hundreds of medical studies about this subject, but basically they all point to the following factors as the major causes of heart disease: diet (eating too much animal fat and being overweight), smoking, lifestyle (too much stress and too little exercise), heredity, and diseases such as hypertension and diabetes.

There's not much that you and I can do about factors like heredity, but there's a lot we can do when it comes to diet,

smoking, and lifestyles! We can eat healthy, nutritious food instead of junk, we can stop smoking, and we can exercise and reduce the stress in our lives! (I hope you were paying particular attention to that second one, 'cause that's something you can do right now!)

Specific Medical Considerations

Most people with heart disease can greatly improve their health with a program of regular exercise. But you should NOT exercise if you have any of the following:

- recent myocardial infarction (The scars from this condition can take up to six weeks to become firm, and until that time exercise can cause a bulging of the scar and a possible aneurysm.)
- acute heart failure
- rapidly progressing anginal pain

- myocarditis (an inflammation of the tissue surrounding the heart)
- an aortic or ventricular aneurysm
- grossly irregular heart action
- recent pulmonary embolism (blood clots in the lungs)
- congenital heart disease
- a fixed-rate pacemaker

Each of these conditions is very complex and it's impossible to discuss them in detail here. Therefore, play it safe and plan your program of exercise only with your physician's approval.

Specific Nutritional Concerns

Diet plays a major role in the prevention and treatment of heart disease. And the primary culprit in an unhealthy diet is animal fat. Did you know that if you are the average American 35 to 40 percent of the calories you eat every day are made up of animal fat?? 35 to 40 percent! I can hear you right now. You're denying it. You cut the fat off your pork chops and you never eat bacon, right? But white bread, cookies, cakes, packaged pastries, gravies, salad dressings, fried chicken, hot dogs, and hamburgers all contain large amounts of animal fat. Your assignment for the day is to reread the chapter on good nutrition.

Warning Signs of Physical Overextension

You should stop exercising if you notice any of the following symptoms: angina (pain in your heart), light-headedness, severe fatigue, nausea, cold moist skin, cyanosis (a bluish tint to the skin), staggering, mental confusion, drooping eyelids, or a severe drop or rise in blood pressure.

If you have heart disease, a regular program of exercise can do lots of great things for your body:

—Exercise will get more blood to your diseased heart and provide it with oxygen and nourishment.

—Exercise will make your heart and blood vessels more efficient.

—Exercise can help to lower blood cholesterol.

—Exercise can lower tension and the other effects of stress.

One final recommendation from the American Heart Association is that your exercise program consist of three stages:

1. Warm-Up (five to ten minutes of stretching and flexing)
2. Exercise (fifteen to thirty minutes of physician-approved exercises)
3. Cool-Down (five to ten minutes of walking or stretching)

HEMOPHILIA

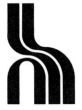

OrthopædicHospital

Consultants:

Stephen J. Snyder, M.D.
—Orthopedic Surgeon
   Southern California Sports Medicine
     and Orthopedic Medical Group
   Van Nuys, CA

Shelby Dietrich, M.D.
—Director
   Hemophilia Center
   Orthopaedic Hospital
   Los Angeles, CA

Consultant:

Alice Lois Boylen, M.D.
—President
   Hemophilia Foundation
     of Southern California
   Los Angeles, CA

Definition

After an injury like a cut or a bruise, blood clotting is the body's normal defense system. The clotted blood stops any further blood loss and actually seals or protects an open wound. This clotting process is caused by the protein Factor VIII. Hemophilia (along with related diseases such as Christmas disease, Von Willebrand's disease, and other platelet deficiencies) is a medical condition that occurs when Factor VIII is either present in very small amounts or totally absent. When bleeding occurs, hemophilia is treated with replacement injections of the missing protein and with instructions on the physical techniques for controlling bleeding (ice, splints, and physical therapy).

I discussed the subject of hemophilia with Dr. Stephen J. Snyder, and he gave me some very specific information you should consider when planning your exercise program.

First, Dr. Snyder told me many of you fear that exercise will cause bleeding. Not the kind of "surface" bleeding most people associate with hemophilia, but the kind of bleeding that can occur deep within the muscle tissue and joints. Aside from causing temporary swelling, pain, and stiffness, bleeding in a joint can have lasting effects. It may, for example, impede the normal growth and development of cartilage surrounding joints. Over a long period, such bleeding may even cause arthritis.

But even at a very young age, you can learn to identify the early warning signs of internalized bleeding. These would include swelling, tightness, a constant or throbbing pain, or numbness (particularly in the arms and legs).

Perhaps the most important thing Dr. Snyder stressed is that there is absolutely no reason for you to be sedentary or immobile. In fact, you *must* exercise. Controlled movement and exercise are essential for rehabilitation of hemophilia. Exercise helps you in two ways:

First, when you do not use your muscles, they become weak and stiff. Then you are more likely to develop other problems, like arthritis.

Second—and this is the really important part—new medical research shows that when you *don't* move you are more likely to experience bleeding deep within your joints. So you're NOT protecting yourself when you move slowly and "sit very still." This kind of inactivity only increases the chances that you *will* bleed.

Specific Medical Considerations

Of course, everybody is an individual. Some of you have a small percentage of clotting substances and some of you have none present in your blood. So naturally, your exercise program must be specific to your needs and approved by your physician. But you can also use your own good common sense. Contact sports such as football, soccer, and boxing are definitely "out" for you. You knew that already, right? But you should also consider your medical history when planning the kinds of activities you can do. If, for example, you have arthritis in your knee, then you shouldn't join the track team or the running club. And if you have experienced bleeding in your shoulder or your elbow, then you shouldn't sign up for tennis lessons.

Common Psychological or Behavioral Barriers to Exercise

You feel left out sometimes, don't you? All of your friends are playing football and you sit on the sidelines with a bag of popcorn. Or maybe you decide to "tough it out"—I mean, after all, you *look* just like everybody out there on the playing field. You just go ahead and do whatever you want, despite the doctors' warnings! But both of these attitudes can cause you big problems, because neither is accepting reality. You won't become the football captain, and worrying about it or denying it only wastes your time and energy. Get busy with what you can do! Keep trim and strong and healthy with a moderate exercise program. It doesn't take much; it just takes planning and consistency. A little exercise every day will keep your body in top condition.

Warning Signs of Physical Overextension

Pay attention to what your body is telling you. If during exercise you feel a tightness or pain in one of your joints, or if you notice any numbness or weakness (particularly in your calves or forearms)— STOP EXERCISING, contact your doctor, and follow your normal procedures for controlling early bleeding.

I asked Dr. Snyder if he had some final thoughts he would like to share with you. And he did:

"The hemophiliac population is, indeed, a very special group of people. And life for this group is full of trade-offs. Often when a person with hemophilia cannot pursue rigorous sporting activities, he has more time to perfect and achieve his chosen vocation. But a good brain and a quick wit will be of no use if they cannot be taken into the courtroom or the executive office by a healthy, well-functioning body. Overall fitness and exercise programs must be started early in life and continued throughout the patient's good times and bad times.

"Close involvement with the physical therapist and physician is important, but the person with hemophilia must learn to maintain his own program of rehabilitation. The responsibility for maintaining motion and muscle tone, hence mobility and extremity use, rests solely upon the individual. The health professionals are there to assist and advise, but motivation must come from within. A person with hemophilia is just a person who bleeds a little more than the average. He is just a 'normal kid with a few bad joints.'"

HYPERTENSION

OrthopædicHospital

Consultant:

Russell Kurihara, M.D.
—Clinical Instructor of Medicine
  University of Southern California
    School of Medicine
  Orthopaedic Hospital
  Los Angeles, CA

Definition

Simply put, hypertension is elevated blood pressure. This rise in pressure comes about because of abnormal resistance to the flow of blood throughout your body. We still don't know all the reasons for such resistance, but doctors suspect elements of diet (including obesity), smoking, hereditary predisposition, emotional stress, and/or illness. It's estimated that about 25 percent of all American adults have some form of hypertension. You can have this condition for years and never know it until you suddenly become ill with symptoms such as fatigue, dizziness, nervousness, sleeplessness, weakness, or headaches. If you don't treat hypertension (both with medication and a change in lifestyle), you will find yourself facing sudden heart failure, stroke, or even death.

A measurement of blood pressure consists of two numbers: for example, 120/80. The first number represents the pressure existing at the instant your heart muscle beats. This is called the "systolic" reading. The second number, or "diastolic" reading, is the pressure present as your heart rests. Generally speaking, normal adult blood pressure ranges from a systolic pressure of 110 to 140, and from a diastolic pressure of 70 to 90.

There is no cure for hypertension, BUT IT CAN BE CONTROLLED with medication, diet, changes in lifestyle, and regular exercise. It's really important that you work to keep your blood pressure within normal limits, and the following lifelong habits will help you do just that:

—Stop smoking.
—Avoid excessive alcohol.
—Keep your weight at a level ideal for your age, height, and activity level.
—Exercise daily.
—Resolve personal conflicts that can lead to stress.
—Practice moderation in all activities,

keeping a balance between work, rest, and recreation.

Specific Medical Considerations

When you begin a program of general exercise, it's essential that you see your doctor first so he or she can evaluate any damage an elevated pressure may have already done to your body. Exercise will cause changes in your blood pressure and may require modifications of your daily medications. Most important, your doctor can teach you how to monitor your own blood pressure and help prevent any complications from overextension.

Specific Nutritional Concerns

Sodium can make it more difficult for your body to remove excess fluids, and so most people with hypertension need to avoid table salt, canned foods, carbonated beverages, and sodium bicarbonate. Please, learn to read labels on processed foods. You'll be amazed at where salt is hiding!

Warning Signs of Physical Overextension

Regular (that means daily) exercise is a MUST for you. And your doctor has probably already included exercise in your treatment plan. But Dr. Russell Kurihara of Orthopaedic Hospital in Los Angeles told me that when you begin exercise (especially if you've been sitting for years) you can expect a gradual increase in your pulse rate and breathing. But if you notice any of the following signs, stop exercising and notify your doctor: chest pain, rapid heartbeat, severe headache, weakness in an arm or a leg, persistent cough, increasing shortness of breath, or dizziness.

Dr. Kurihara had these final words for you: "Make certain that you have a physical checkup. Then start an exercise program that involves a sport or routine you thoroughly enjoy. Begin slowly and gradually increase the duration and intensity of the workouts."

IDIOPATHIC SCOLIOSIS

OrthopædicHospital

Consultants:

Robert Gustafson, M.D.
And The Scoliosis Committee of
  Orthopaedic Hospital:
  Carol Alford, M.S.W., L.C.S.W.
  Agatha Jones, L.V.N.

Lynne Morihisa, R.P.T., B.S.
Kathryn Smith, R.N., M.N.
Sandra Stuckey, R.P.T., M.A.
Patricia Torres, R.N., B.S.
Rosemary Treiger Van Gorder, M.A.
Los Angeles, CA

Definition

Scoliosis, more commonly known as "curvature of the spine," is a lateral (side-to-side) deviation in the alignment of the spinal vertebrae. In a small percentage of people, the spine curves sideward because of some illness affecting muscles of the back (as in polio), and, occasionally, the spine curvature occurs during fetal development. (The latter is called congenital scoliosis.) However, in the vast majority of cases the cause is still unknown. This condition is called idiopathic scoliosis.

Idiopathic scoliosis affects about 5 to 10 percent of all adolescents, becoming most apparent during periods of rapid growth. Usually, it involves no pain and appears first in very subtle ways, such as one hip that seems slightly higher or one shoulder blade that is somewhat more prominent. Besides being subtle, these changes can often be hidden by clothing or poor posture. Thus, scoliosis can come as a complete shock to both child and parent. For this reason, many states are now including scoliosis screening in the health examinations of schoolchildren.

Because the curvature usually worsens with periods of growth, a child with scoliosis must be monitored very closely by a physician. Often, the curvature stops and remains as a minor misalignment. In these cases, people may lead fully functional lives with little or no discomfort. In other cases, however, the vertebrae will continue "to move sideward," eventually causing severe back pain, difficulty with breathing, and/or heart problems. And so monitoring the movement of the vertebrae by physical examination and X ray determines the course of proper treatment.

Specific Medical Considerations

For many years, medical information regarding this condition was somewhat stable. But Dr. Robert Gustafson of Orthopaedic Hospital in Los Angeles tells me that new theories and techniques in the treatment of scoliosis are now being developed very rapidly. Currently, the first course of treatment is observation (to see if the condition worsens or stabilizes). The second step is the use of a back brace, and the third is corrective surgery.

It's important for you to realize that exercise will not stop the progression of scoliosis. But, particularly when a child is wearing a brace, stretching exercises can increase flexibility and keep his or her back muscles from becoming rigid. And in more advanced cases, exercise can occasionally help reduce back pain.

Common Psychological or Behavioral Barriers to Exercise

Scoliosis is frequently discovered during adolescence, a time when lots of important changes are taking place. But successful treatment (braces and orthopedic surgery after your growth has stabilized) can give you a bright and hopeful future, full of all kinds of activities.

Specific Precautions for a Program of General Exercise

If you have scoliosis, you must avoid heavy weight lifting, tumbling, and movement on equipment such as a trampoline.

The best kinds of exercises for you may be extension (backward bending of the trunk) for the upper spine and flexion (forward bending of the trunk) for the lower spine. Some examples of extension exercises are CSH 3 Superkid (page 168) and CWS 5 Airplane (page 185). Examples of flexion exercises are CWS 3 Your Majesty (page 186) and CWS 6 Pelvic Tilt (page 190).

It's recommended that you exercise two times daily, once in the morning and once at night. A good starting point would be twenty repetitions of each exercise.

Remember, after treatment most people with scoliosis are able to lead active lives, including regular exercise and participation in most sports.

MALIGNANT BONE TUMOR

Orthopædic*Hospital*

Consultant:

Nadia Ewing, M.D.
—Codirector of the California Children's
    Service Tumor Center
  Orthopaedic Hospital
  Los Angeles, CA

Definition

Malignant bone tumors are defined as abnormal growths of rapidly multiplying cells, which in turn destroy normal bone tissue. In addition, these tumors can spread to other parts of the body. They are a relatively rare yet quite serious form of cancer in children. The cause of bone cancer is unknown, but there is speculation that it may be caused by chemicals, radiation, viruses, or an inherited predisposition. (Please, also read the general appendix entry titled "Cancer.")

Specific Medical Considerations

Medical considerations are based primarily upon a person's general health and reactions to treatment of the cancer. There are three major forms of treatment for someone with bone cancer: surgery, radiation therapy, or chemotherapy. Surgery may include either limb salvage or amputation. (If appropriate for you or your child, please note the appendix entry regarding amputation.) Radiation therapy may cause shrinking of the muscle mass overlying the affected bone and a consequential loss of function and range of motion of adjacent joints. The side effects of chemotherapy can include both emotional and physical reactions. There may be weakness, anemia, and increased susceptibility to infection. Because each of these may affect your exercise program, it's essential that you check with your doctor before beginning.

Common Psychological or Behavioral Barriers to Exercise

It's scary enough just being in the hospital, and sometimes the treatment for your cancer can add to your anxiety. You may, for example, have to face the trauma of amputation and then lose your hair because of chemotherapy. Particularly if you're a teenager, losing your hair can be devastating. This is where planning and practicing regular exercise can help. Suddenly, you can get control over a part of your life again instead of just having people do things *to* you.

Specific Precautions for a Program of General Exercise

Dr. Nadia Ewing, a pediatric hematologist/oncologist, told me that specific precautions should be handled on an individual basis by your own doctor. "For example," she said, "radiation therapy can weaken some bones and so jumping or jolting could easily cause a fracture. Or, a patient who is anemic because of chemotherapy might easily become short of breath, and therefore be unable to perform more vigorous forms of exercise."

Dr. Ewing also told me that depending upon the individual, isometric exercises and activities such as swimming and bicycling can be excellent ways to begin your lifelong program of exercise.

She concluded, "Take good care of yourself; you're worth the effort. Staying in shape is healthy and it makes you look terrific!"

MULTIPLE SCLEROSIS

Consultants:

Audrey Spiegel Goldman, M.A.
—Chapter Services Director
  National Multiple Sclerosis Society
  Southern California Chapter
  Glendale, CA

Linda Lawson, R.P.T.
—Chairperson
  Chapter Services Committee
  National Multiple Sclerosis Society
  Southern California Chapter
  Glendale, CA

Consultant:

Debra Frankel
—Director
  Support Services
  National Multiple Sclerosis Society
  Massachusetts Chapter
  Waltham, MA
—Co-author with
    Robert Buxbaum, M.D.,
    Maximizing Your Health

Definition

We don't yet know what causes multiple sclerosis (MS), but we do know how it affects people. Throughout all of our bodies, there is a vast neurological network carrying messages to and from the brain. MS attacks the myelin sheath (a coating and insulation) surrounding message-carrying nerve fibers in the brain and spinal cord. When myelin is destroyed, it is replaced by hardened tissue or plaque (sclerosis). Both the hardened material and the damaged myelin areas will then interfere with the transmission of neurological signals. With mild MS, the nerve impulses can still be transmitted, but with minor interruptions. Later, if the disease progresses, the sclerosis can completely obstruct messages your brain sends to other parts of your body.

Because different areas of the brain and spinal cord can be affected in varying amounts, each person experiences MS in a different way. You may experience a series of attacks and then find that the disease is in partial or even complete remission. Or you may experience a gradual and steady worsening of symptoms. Some of the more common symptoms seen in the disease are general weakness, tingling, numbness, impaired sensation, lack of coordination, disturbances in equilibrium, double vision, involuntary and rapid movement of the eyes, slurred speech, tremor, stiffness or spasticity, fatigue, and bladder problems. In more severe cases, you may even experience total paralysis of the extremities.

Common Psychological or Behavioral Barriers to Exercise

Debra Frankel, director of Support Services for the Massachusetts Chapter of the National Multiple Sclerosis Society, referred to the unpredictability of MS when she told me of some of the common psychological problems associated with the disease. Because MS can often "come and go," with bouts of severe attacks and then remission, and because the symptoms are so variable, it's a challenge for you to maintain a good, strong positive attitude. As soon as you think you've got it all under control, another attack of muscle weakness, numbness, or even paralysis seems to pop out of nowhere. This is where a regular pattern of exercise may help combat depression. The routine is the key. It doesn't matter if some days you can't do all of the exercises or all of the repetitions. Just do your best. Keep to the routine. And every time you can complete the exercise—or even add another exercise—celebrate each triumph, 'cause you're doing something good for yourself!

Specific Precautions for a Program of General Exercise

Fatigue and overheating can sometimes worsen the symptoms of MS, and so it's very important that you pay attention to the signals from your own body. Particularly if you have not exercised for a long time, pace yourself. Start slowly and add exercises as you increase your stamina. The National Multiple Sclerosis Society suggests dividing your time into four equal periods of "exercise-rest-exercise-rest."

Finally, since many people with MS often experience difficulty with balance, you need to be cautious during any exercise requiring this skill. (Exercises requiring good balance are those in which you have to stand on one foot or stand with your feet close together.)

Warning Signs of Physical Overextension

In addition to fatigue and overheating, you should be aware of any increase in spasticity or tremors, pain, any dizziness or loss of balance, or any generalized feelings of stress or anxiety.

Linda Lawson ended our conversation with a beautiful thought that seems appropriate to *any* handicapable person: "Every person has the ultimate responsibility for his or her own health. An individual with Multiple Sclerosis must maintain hope and belief for a cure, and in the meantime, strive to achieve and maintain a balanced, active and worthwhile lifestyle. To quote Molly Mizrahi, a woman with MS, 'I don't know when there will be a cure—but I want to be ready.' "

MUSCULAR DYSTROPHY

OrthopædicHospital

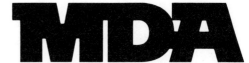

Consultant:

Robert Wiedbusch, M.D.
   Orthopaedic Hospital
   Los Angeles,CA

Consultant:

Rodney E. Brandon
—Patient Service Coordinator
   Muscular Dystrophy Association
   New York, NY

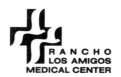

Consultant:

Antje K. Hunt, M.S., R.P.T.
—Equipment Consultant
   Rancho Los Amigos Medical Center
   Downey, CA

Definition

Muscular dystrophy is a group of neuro-muscular diseases characterized by a wasting away and progressive weakness of the skeletal muscles. While the condition can strike anyone of any age, almost all of its victims are children.

The most common variety is Duchenne Muscular Dystrophy, an inherited disability seen almost exclusively in young boys. (It is theoretically possible, but extremely rare, for the disease to be seen in girls. Rather, the gene conveying DMD is normally carried by a female and then transmitted to her son.)

New information about the course of this disease reminds us always to think of each person as an individual, but the disorder usually follows the same pattern. As an infant, the child with DMD may look and act perfectly normal. But as he begins to walk, his family can notice signs of muscle weakness such as frequent falling, difficulty in standing, and movement often dismissed as clumsiness. Exercise, physical therapy, and braces can sometimes delay the muscle deterioration (especially when the child remains ambulatory and able to walk). But by early adolescence, many children with DMD find it necessary to use a wheelchair. (Many of our exercises for children may be done while seated.)

Specific Precautions for a Program of General Exercise

Children who are still ambulatory often have trouble with balance. Therefore, it may be advisable for your child to use protective headgear when he or she is exercising.

Warning Signs of Physical Overextension

Dr. Wiedbusch suggests that you watch for excessive sweating, rapid pulse or breathing, or a sudden loss of remaining muscle strength. If any of these conditions occurs, you should stop the exercise program and contact your physician.

The kinds of exercises most beneficial to a child with muscular dystrophy are those that move his joints through their normal range of motion, and breathing exercises that utilize the chest wall and the diaphragm.

Antje Hunt, a physical therapist with Rancho Los Amigos Medical Center, had these fantastic suggestions for your exercise program: "Concentrate upon competition with yourself, not with relatively more able-bodied children. For more fun and variety, try exercising in different positions, different environments and *with other people.* Turn your *routine* into an *exercise potpourri.*

"If exercise is not possible at all, you can still 'work out' with an electric wheelchair as you *dance* to music. Or ask someone to tie a baseball bat to the footrest of your wheelchair so you can *kick* a basketball or soccer ball around a gym or a yard. Make a game of it as you try to get the ball into the opponent's goal. It'll make the adrenaline flow and cause as much huffing and puffing as in a championship soccer match!"

And our experts had something to say to you parents: Many activities will not be possible for a child with a progressive disease like muscular dystrophy. This is why it's especially important that you encourage him to tackle those physical tasks he can do. A regular program of exercise and movement is one such challenge. Your child is probably already involved in an extensive program of physical therapy in which his muscles are moved and stretched to delay the onset of muscle contractures. And while an additional exercise program will not halt or cure his condition, it can give him something else of great value. It can give him something to achieve. Because he must rely upon you and health professionals for so much, this is a healthful way for him to develop independence and enjoy his own accomplishment. Allow *him* to plan his exercise program, present it to the doctor and therapist, and have total responsibility for its daily execution.

Antje had these final words for your child: "Exercise is a mood lifter. Be positive and creative in your exercise plan; adapt exercises to fit your abilities and needs. If you exercise regularly, the quality of your life will improve and your 'struggle' with muscular dystrophy will become easier. Don't *allow* a muscle disease to 'handicap' you!"

OSTEOGENESIS IMPERFECTA

OrthopædicHospital

Consultants:

Shelby Deitrich, M.D.

Kathryn Horn, R.P.T.
—Physical Therapist

Michael Pantiel, M.S.W.
—Social Worker
  Orthopaedic Hospital
  Los Angeles, CA

Definition

Osteogenesis imperfecta (OI) is a rare, multifaceted genetic disease of the connective tissue of the body. It's commonly called the "brittle bone disease" because people with OI are very prone to fractures of their long bones. (In fact, some people may have over 200 fractures in a lifetime.) There are varying degrees of OI, ranging from very mild to very severe. In addition to bone fractures, the most severe forms of the disease can present the following challenges: hearing loss, dental and skeletal malformations (often including scoliosis), joint hypermobility (looseness), and short stature.

Specific Medical Considerations

Without a doubt, fractures are the major concern when you have OI. You must exercise regularly to maintain muscle tone and joint health, but each exercise must be carefully planned so as not to risk breaking a bone. The second major orthopedic challenge you face is scoliosis (curvature of the spine), and here, too, you and your doctor must determine which exercises will be best for you.

If you have OI, you may also experience many more respiratory infections (you've really got to watch those flu epidemics), other cardiopulmonary diseases, diaphoresis (an excessive amount of perspiration), and a higher incidence of hernias.

Common Psychological or Behavioral Barriers to Exercise

Michael Pantiel, a social worker with Orthopaedic Hospital in Los Angeles, told me that the fear of fractures is quite significant in your life. And as a result, parents and friends of a person with OI very often become overprotective. You sometimes have to fight very hard to maintain your independence. Having an altered body image can also make it difficult to maintain your self-esteem.

That's why it's essential to concentrate on your intellectual and emotional strengths. You've spent a lot of time with doctors and other health professionals— you know more than anyone else how important good nutrition and regular, *appropriate* exercise can be for you. Cardiopulmonary disease is the most common cause of death for a person with OI, and exercise and diet are major elements in its prevention.

Specific Nutritional Concerns

The same diaphoresis that produces excessive perspiration and the fact that you may be inactive can both lead to chronic constipation. In order to combat this problem, you should eat a well-balanced diet including lots of fresh fruits, vegetables, and grains. And especially during warm weather or after exercise, increase your consumption of liquids. Your doctor or a nutritionist can give you the specifics for your body size and overall condition.

Specific Precautions for a Program of General Exercise

First and foremost, avoid any exercise that may increase your chances of a fracture. Depending upon the degree of OI, you should avoid any exercise that includes jogging, jumping, bouncing, twisting (especially your head), applying pressure to limbs, pushing, pulling, or bending.

Instead, you should use slow, methodical movements such as those seen in the stretching and relaxation exercises in chapters Three and Five. Deep breathing exercises can be done in a seated position and will help maintain good pulmonary function. And because it is a non-weight-bearing activity, swimming may be a very good exercise for you.

Most of all, you should proceed slowly and use your own good common sense. Don't let anybody talk you out of it. If you and your doctor plan appropriate exercises and if you observe some basic cautions, you can also make exercise a fun and valuable part of your life.

OSTEOPOROSIS

OrthopædicHospital

Consultant:

Charles F. Sharp, Jr., M.D.
—Associate Professor of Clinical
    Medicine
   University of Southern California
   School of Medicine

—Director
   Osteoporosis Treatment Center
   Orthopaedic Hospital
   Los Angeles, CA

Definition

When I talk with silver citizens about exercise, they often confide a fear of bone fractures. It seems that most of us know of somebody who experienced a hip or an arm fracture after a relatively slight fall. Most of the time these kinds of fractures happen because of a condition known as osteoporosis. This is a decrease in bone mass caused by factors such as hormonal changes brought about by menopause in women (25 percent of women over the age of sixty have this condition!), nutritional imbalance (like too little calcium), other diseases, and physical inactivity.

But if you have osteoporosis, there is no reason to fear exercise. In fact, you need it just like everybody else. And with planning and consistency, you can develop an exercise program that can actually help increase the density of your bone mass and decrease the chance of a fracture.

Specific Medical Considerations

Dr. Charles F. Sharp, a specialist in the treatment of osteoporosis, tells me that the medical limitations of your exercise program depend very much upon where and how often you have experienced a bone fracture. Fractures of the wrist and proximal forearm, for example, usually heal very well and mean only a moderate limitation of your exercise program. Fractures of the vertebral spine, however, can lead to a chronic back pain that may place more limits on the amount of exercise time and the types of exercises you can follow. The most severe type of fracture, Dr. Sharp says, is a fracture of the hip. In this instance, you may need surgery, a long-term hospital stay, and physical therapy and rehabilitation. In all cases, you should clear any exercise plan with your physician.

Common Psychological or Behavioral Barriers to Exercise

Dr. Sharp says that after learning of osteoporosis you may look at yourself "as though old age had abruptly taken over a previously young and healthy body." In other words, you give up. You decide that you're old and that old people need to sit and rock on the front porch. I don't mean any disrespect, but you are WRONG, WRONG, WRONG. Everybody gets old; some of us are just better at it than others.

Then there is the justifiable fear of falling. Sometimes this can occupy every waking moment. It can even cause you to have nightmares! But if you begin exercising slowly, observe the common sense rules of safety, and build your program only as your strength increases, then your chances of falling are greatly reduced. And, Dr. Sharp adds, "In my experience, once the patient has begun to exercise, a fear of falling often recedes."

Specific Nutritional Concerns

You need lots more calcium—as much as 1,000 milligrams a day if you are a premenopausal woman (or if you take estrogen), and as much as 1,500 milligrams a day if you are postmenopausal. Your physician may prescribe calcium or other supplements, such as magnesium, zinc, and vitamin D.

Also, it is important for you to severely limit caffeine and alcohol and to stop smoking. (See—everybody is very serious about this caffeine, alcohol, and smoking business!)

Finally, avoid fad diets (especially those that tell you to eat lots of protein or carbohydrates).

Specific Precautions for a Program of General Exercise

Remember that the dangers of *immobilization* can be just as important to you now. You need to keep active if you're to keep healthy! But the specifics of your exercise program must be planned around other medical factors that may accompany osteoporosis and aging. So check with your physician if you have any other cardiovascular, pulmonary, musculoskeletal, or neurological diseases.

If you have had a spinal fracture, strenuous lifting of even small weights may be dangerous, and, again, you should observe safety rules (like not exercising on a loose rug or near furniture).

Specifically, sit-ups or spinal exercises (such as bending at the waist) may be quite desirable for a younger person without manifested spinal fracture, but if you have spinal osteoporosis, DO NOT do these exercises.

Jogging and striking exercises (like jumping jacks) must be avoided if you have a severe loss in bone density. But younger patients who have not yet developed severe loss should participate in as many of these weight-bearing exercises as is tolerable. (That sounds a little confusing, at first. But, obviously, this judgment must be made with the help of your physician.)

Finally, Dr. Sharp recommends walking as an excellent way to begin your exercise program.

Warning Signs of Physical Overextension

If you have spinal osteoporosis, you should stop exercising if you feel an increase in back pain.

Most often, however, a fracture—the end point for osteoporotic bone—cannot be predicted. Your best plan is a slow, steady exercise program that can gradually increase your strength and decrease the chance of fracture.

Dr. Sharp had some very interesting comments on this last point: "Bone is a dynamic tissue which responds to stress at all times during life. That stress which is induced by exercise, if done in the proper fashion, can increase bone density just as muscle mass is increased. My only qualification is that this exercise must be performed on a regular basis. And if possible should consist of thirty minutes of vigorous exercise five times a week."

OSTOMY

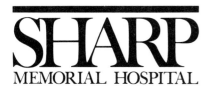

MEMORIAL HOSPITAL

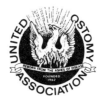

Consultant:

Linda L. Bauer, R.N.
—Staff Nurse
  Sharp Memorial Hospital
  San Diego, CA

Consultants:

Donald P. Binder
—Director

Katherine F. Jeter, Ed.D., E.T.
—Enterostomal Therapist
  United Ostomy Association
  Los Angeles, CA

Definition

An ostomy is a surgically created opening in the abdominal wall. It's constructed to serve as either a permanent or temporary passageway for the disposal of waste products (urine or feces). The reasons for such surgery are many, but some of the more common are inflammatory bowel disease, ulcerative colitis, congenital defects in the digestive system, cancer, and severe injury. The important thing to remember about an ostomy is that it bypasses damaged, diseased, or even removed digestive organs and thus makes you healthy again.

The three most common forms of ostomy are the colostomy (an opening from the colon or large intestine), the ileostomy (an opening from the small intestine, usually after the large intestine has been removed), and the urostomy (a general term for any opening from the urinary system).

The actual opening of an ostomy is created by bringing a portion of the intestine or urinary tract to the surface of your body, and this is called the "stoma." While the stoma requires some maintenance and the use of a pouch or an appliance to collect waste materials, it is also what keeps your body functioning. Before you leave the hospital, you'll be taught maintenance techniques for the stoma, and once the surgery has healed, you should be able to return to all of your normal activities. In fact, most people usually feel better than they have for years.

Specific Medical Considerations

People with ostomies run marathons, climb mountains, and do almost anything else they want. But if you have had an ostomy, you must remember that abdominal surgery takes some time to heal. So you must check with your physician before beginning any kind of exercise program.

Common Psychological or Behavioral Barriers to Exercise

Your most difficult problem may be the psychological obstacle of altered body image. Suddenly, you're "different." More than that, you may feel uncomfortable discussing your difference with others. Society is partly to blame, because even though we openly discuss mastectomy, birth control, and every other kind of surgery, somehow people still seem embarrassed about surgery of the bowel or urinary system. Your biggest concerns are over the practical matters: "Will the appliance show under my clothing?" "Will I have an accident and leakage?" "What about odor?" But usually, no one will know about your ostomy unless you choose to tell them.

When you exercise, it's a good idea for you to play it safe and carry along extra supplies for your appliance. But otherwise, you have very few restrictions to a normal, active life. The important thing for you to remember is that regular exercise and good nutrition are fantastic ways to build your confidence and decrease stress or anxiety. Once you get going, you'll wonder why you ever worried about it in the first place.

Specific Nutritional Concerns

Most individuals with an ostomy need only follow the same FOOD 4 LIFE plan discussed in Chapter Four, but Linda Bauer, R.N., with Memorial Sloan-Kettering Cancer Center did give me a few examples of specialized diets you *may* require at some time in your rehabilitation:

—When your surgery has involved removal of the large bowel, you may have to increase your intake of potassium. (Good foods for this are bananas, oranges, prunes, and tomatoes.)

—Some people with ileostomies require supplemental B12 vitamins.

—When you have had any kind of ostomy, you probably will need to drink much more water.

—You will need to concentrate on those foods that help prevent constipation. (These include high-residue and high-fiber foods like fruit, bran, whole grains, and vegetables. The one exception to a high-fiber diet may be if you have an ileostomy.)

—Many people with ileostomies and some with colostomies need to avoid foods high in cellulose. (These would include popcorn, celery strings, coconut, shells of peas, bamboo shoots, and bean sprouts.)

—When diarrhea occurs, replace normal fluids with bouillon, tea with a little sugar, ginger ale, or Gatorade. Foods to eat when you have a problem with diarrhea include rice, crackers, bananas, potatoes, and cheese.

—Maybe of most importance to you is the prevention of gas. (The muscles that normally regulate the release of gas probably will have been removed.) This is an individual matter, but some foods that produce gas in most people are cabbage, onions, cucumbers, beans, melons, and refined sugars. You can also help prevent gas by eating your meals slowly and avoiding chewing gum (which causes you to swallow excess air).

These are just general suggestions; you'll need to discuss the specifics of your diet and body with your doctor or nutritonist.

Specific Precautions for a Program of General Exercise

If you've just had surgery, your abdominal muscles must be sufficiently healed before beginning any exercise, so check with your doctor first. Otherwise, your only precautions would fall in the "good sense" category: Avoid any hard contact to your stoma; don't do any heavy lifting (you definitely do not need a hernia right now!); and begin slowly, building up your exercise program as you improve.

Warning Signs of Physical Overextension

You need to look out for the signs of excessive perspiration loss. These include weakness, thirst, muscle cramping, and decreased urine output. If you are losing too much perspiration, you've got to replace fluids immediately. Liquids such as Gatorade may help replace needed electrolytes, and Linda Bauer recommends the following "quick toddy": 1 tsp. salt, 1 tsp. baking soda, 4 tsps. white Karo syrup, 1 6-oz. can frozen orange juice. Drink one half cup every hour. Shortly after your first drink, call your doctor!

I asked Linda and Katherine Jeter, of the United Ostomy Association, if they had any final words for you and they did. Katherine told me, "An ostomy is for living and living is more fun and more satisfying when people are in good physical condition. Follow the example of people with ostomies who golf, swim, run and dance—be well, be fit."

Linda added, "If you have an ostomy you will initially face tremendous physical and psychological hurdles. Yet with proper instruction, understanding and support, the hurdles can be cleared. Once you recognize your ostomy as a liberation from disease, you'll find few restrictions to your lifestyle. After all, Babe Didrickson Zacharias won the 1954 Women's U.S. Open Golf Championship— one year after her colostomy for cancer."

PARKINSON'S DISEASE
(Parkinson's Syndrome)

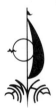

Consultants:

Bill Cox, R.P.T.
—Director of Rehabilitation Services
  Hoag Memorial Hospital Presbyterian
—Coordinator Parkinson's Information
  Exchange

Janet Chance, M.D.
—Medical Advisor

Sheila Gilmore, M.A., C.C.C.
—Speech Pathologist

Fred Meister, Ph.D.
—Clinical Pharmacologist

Donna Bayhan, R.P.T.
—Therapist

Candace Simonds, O.T.R.
—Therapist
  Parkinson's Information Exchange
  Hoag Memorial Hospital Presbyterian
  Newport Beach, CA

Definition

Our muscles and the nerves that regulate them work because of a very complex system of chemical and electrical action and reaction. Dopamine, a chemical released by certain cells in your brain, is one vital element in this system. Parkinson's disease results from a disorder of those brain cells that regulate the release of dopamine. The effects of Parkinson's vary from person to person, but they usually include muscle tremor or shaking, a slowness of movement, difficulty in initiating movement, rigidity or stiffness, a shuffling walk, and problems with speech and/or swallowing. The loss of automatic muscle responses means that if you have Parkinson's disease you probably need to make a concentrated effort to move certain muscles.

Specific Medical Considerations

Sometimes Parkinson's disease can cause dizziness and light-headedness. If this is true for you, concentrate on those exercises in which you can be seated or in which you can brace yourself with a wall or piece of furniture.

Common Psychological or Behavioral Barriers to Exercise

When anyone has a problem with movement and/or communication, the "normal" psychological reaction is usually depression and withdrawal. You have to *fight* to stay active and involved because sometimes it's so easy *just to give up.* And Parkinson's, like so many other neuromuscular diseases, can have "on-again, off-again" symptoms. You may not know when a symptom will occur, and you most certainly hate the idea of becoming increasingly dependent upon your family and friends. Even the medication you take to control the symptoms of your disease can cause memory loss and depression. But Bill Cox, the director of the Parkinson's Information Exchange of Hoag Memorial Hospital, tells me that this is where a regular program of exercise can help. "The more active you are, the more active you can remain," Bill says. "Giving in to the *psychological fallout* from Parkinson's will only result in greater dependency and loss of function."

Specific Nutritional Concerns

Guess what? Your nutritional concerns are just like everybody else's. You get to eat all of the good stuff we discussed in the FOOD 4 LIFE program. There's only one additional precaution. *Everybody's* body works better without caffeine and alcohol, but it's especially important that you avoid them if you've got Parkinson's disease. This is because both chemicals can interfere with muscle control and the absorption of some of your medications. Finally, your pharmacist has probably already told you how B6 vitamin supplements can counteract the effects of dopamine-producing medications.

Specific Precautions for a Program of General Exercise

It's important to observe the same precautions that everyone else does—things like checking with your doctor before beginning your program and approach-ing exercise with a smooth, steady pace instead of a three-minute dash to the Exercise Hall of Fame. Bill and the other consultants from Hoag Memorial suggested some specific movements that might give you the best start:

- Large, smooth movements that emphasize joint flexibility and motion. Examples would be things like raising your arms overhead, and fully bending and straightening your joints (like knees, elbows, and fingers).
- exercises that emphasize and increase your awareness of erect posture
- reciprocal exercises (That means repetitive, alternating large movements, like cycling, swimming, and pool exercises.)
- Daily walks. Pay particular attention to picking up your feet, swinging your arms, and breathing deeply. (Don't forget to look at the birds and smell the flowers. That helps a lot, too!!)
- exercises like trunk rotations that increase the flexibility of your spine and neck
- taking deep breaths and counting out loud when exercising. When you do this, exaggerate the enunciation to exercise the muscles necessary for speech also.

Remember that old saying, "If you don't use it, you'll lose it"? That's particularly true for the person with Parkinson's disease. If you don't use your muscles and joints, they become stiffer, tighter, and less functional. But even more important, exercise makes things easier for you. Because of your disease, you have to work especially hard to control lots of otherwise "automatic" movements. The neuromuscular repetitions in a regular exercise program will make this job easier. You'll be more in control. And you know that anything that gives you more control also makes you feel better.

POLIOMYELITIS AND ADULT POLIO SYNDROME

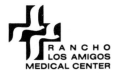

R A N C H O
LOS AMIGOS
MEDICAL CENTER

Consultant:

Jacquelin Perry, M.D.
—Chief
  Pathokinesiology Service
  Rancho Los Amigos Hospital
  Downey, CA
—Professor of Orthopaedics
  University of Southern California
    School of Medicine
  Los Angeles, CA

POLIO SURVIVORS ASSOCIATION

12720 La Reina Ave, Downey, Calif, 90242

Consultant:

Richard Daggett
—President
  Polio Survivors Association
  Downey, CA

Definition

Most people think polio is a thing of the past. And thank God, research and technology have almost wiped out this deadly disease. But there are still thousands of people who having survived polio thirty or more years ago are now experiencing renewed problems with movement. This condition may be called "the postpolio syndrome" or "the late effects of polio." Regardless of the name, the pattern of the problem seems the same. An original polio virus had two effects on the muscles it attacked: Some of the nerves supplying the muscle fibers were destroyed, while others were only temporarily injured. While injured nerves may have recovered, the final result was still a muscle with less than true normal strength. But the human body is an amazing work of engineering and art, and so stronger muscles often took over the work of damaged tissue. This fact was to become important as many polio

survivors regained effective functioning and resumed normal (or even physically active) lives. Doctors, like Jacquelin Perry, are now finding a number of people who have *overworked* their partially recovered muscles. And as a result, these muscles are now beginning to *wear out.*

Specific Medical Considerations

Some doctors ban all exercise for a person experiencing postpolio syndrome. Others, like Dr. Perry, feel that you *can* exercise the rest of your body if you do it with planning and common sense.

It gets a little complicated, but there are some basic dos and don'ts for you.

DON'T exercise polio-affected muscles. Any stress to these now *overworked* muscles can cause a great deal of harm.

DON'T practice stretching exercises until you have had a clinical evaluation from your physician or physical therapist.

289

Sometimes muscle tightness can be a substitute for a lack of direct muscle strength. (It's another way your body has compensated for muscle weakness.) Stretching these muscles can undo such a benefit, and as a result you would have less function than you did before the exercise. The clinical evaluation will determine if the tightness you feel is of an obstructive or a beneficial variety.

DON'T use any exercise (or equipment) that is intended to *power-build* or *strengthen* your muscles. Some examples of strengthening exercises are using weights, aerobics, jogging, and even just doing exercises that require you to lift your body weight when you muscles are too weak to do it spontaneously. Dr. Perry suggested that you do only those exercises and activities that can be done without discomfort. The athlete's philosophy of "no pain, no gain" is totally inappropriate if you already have a disability or a high sensitivity to strain. She reminded me that even athletes later pay penalties for joint and muscle damage done in the name of *sport.*

DON'T give up on exercise completely.

DO, DO, DO exercise the rest of your body. Those muscles that were not affected by the disease and your cardiopulmonary system (your heart and lungs) need normal daily exercise if you are to keep in top condition.

Common Psychological or Behavioral Barriers to Exercise

I know how hard you have to fight being disheartened. After many years of successfully "conquering polio," it's hard to accept the loss of muscle function now. It doesn't seem fair because you've worked so hard to have a normal—maybe even superactive—life. All of those fantastic qualities that got you through your initial recovery—your strength of will, your determination, and your spirit—these very qualities make you want to push on. To fight and to work even harder. The doctors say that physical work—forcing yourself to use your damaged muscles—can have a very negative effect. And I know that this must be hard to hear. But concentrate instead on the kinds of movements you *can* pursue. Simple stretching and even relaxation exercises can help you maintain your body at its peak.

Specific Precautions for a Program of General Exercise

If you are a postpolio patient who has not experienced any of the symptoms described earlier—if you have noticed no muscle weakness in those muscles that have been taking on extra work over the years—you still need to approach exercise with caution. Not fear! But caution. Begin slowly, concentrate on simple stretching and range of motion exercises. Do only those exercises and activities that can be done without discomfort, and pay attention to the warning signs of overextension.

Warning Signs of Physical Overextension

Dr. Perry told me that you must watch very carefully for the following signs: persistent muscle soreness or cramping after the first few days of any new activity, prolonged fatigue, or any evidence of a loss of muscle strength rather than of improvement. If you note any of these conditions, the exercise should be stopped as it could be causing harm or injury to your polio-affected muscles.

PRADER-WILLI SYNDROME

Consultant:

Marge A. Wett
—Executive Director
  Prader-Willi Syndrome Association
  Edina, MN

Definition

The Prader-Willi syndrome is a complex, multisystem disorder that is present at birth. The cause and cure for Prader-Willi have not yet been found, and existing drugs have not yet solved any of the challenges facing children with this syndrome. An infant with Prader-Willi displays a severe lack of muscle development (including even those muscles necessary for the sucking reflex), a failure to thrive because of weakness, and in some cases little sexual development. During childhood, additional symptoms usually appear, and these include developmental delay in the areas of walking and talking, obesity due to a seemingly insatiable appetite, intellectual delays, and behavioral maladjustments. Later symptoms include small hands and feet, short stature, and a delay in or lack of puberty and sexual development.

If your child has Prader-Willi, your physician has undoubtedly told you of the importance of a program of regular physical activity, including therapy and at-home exercise. You will be instructed to provide passive movements several times a day for your child's limbs and head. This form of exercise is essential for building the message pathways from your child's brain to his muscles. Later, as your child develops, you can and should increase exercise periods to his or her fullest potential.

Specific Medical Considerations

A lack of muscle tissue (hypotonia) can improve with time, but your child will experience severe challenge when attempting the usual activities of childhood. A lack of balance, muscle weakness, possible joint complications, and often obesity may limit his or her ability to ride a bicycle, participate in competitive sports and games, run, and have the stamina for rigorous exercise. But a progressive and regular program of general exercise (such as that seen in Chapter Five) and swimming are realistic goals.

Specific Nutritional Concerns

Because children with Prader-Willi can gain weight on half the normal caloric intake, obesity is quite common. Sweets, snacks, and other useless calories are something your child cannot afford, and so most physicians recommend early nutritional education, a diet of less than 1,000 calories a day, and regular exercise.

Specific Precautions for a Program of General Exercise

Marge Wett, executive director of the Prader-Willi Syndrome Association, told me that the best precaution is a complete understanding of your child's abilities and physical challenges. Start slowly with only a few exercises and gradually add activity as your child's skill, confidence, and endurance increase.

Because of difficulties with balance and coordination, people with Prader-Willi are advised to avoid running or jogging and to focus instead on the kinds of slow, stretching exercises seen in chapters Three and Five.

Warning Signs of Physical Overextension

All children should be supervised when they exercise, and your child is no different. Begin slowly and alternate brief activities with rest periods. Stop exercising if your child experiences dizziness, severe pain or cramping, a rapid or irregular heartrate, shortness of breath, or nausea.

Finally, Marge told me, "Exercise must become a regular part of your child's life, but you can turn him against it if *you* expect him to 'keep up' with his peers. Children with Prader-Willi need additional time, practice and encouragement before they can expect to participate in 'normal' activities."

RENAL DISEASE

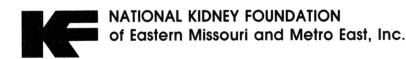

NATIONAL KIDNEY FOUNDATION
of Eastern Missouri and Metro East, Inc.

Consultants:

Sue Caine
—Executive Director

Consultants:

Susan M. Jaskula, M.S.W.
—Renal Social Worker
   St. Louis Regional Dialysis
      Center, Inc.
   St. Louis, MO

Vicky Johnson Stringer, M.S.W.
—Renal Social Worker
   St. Louis Regional Dialysis
      Center, Inc.
   St. Louis, MO

Wendy Weinstock Brown, M.D.
—Chairman Scientific Advisory Board
   National Kidney Foundation of Eastern
      Missouri & Metro East, Inc.
   St. Louis, MO

Sallie E. Taylor, M.Ed., O.T.R.
—Clinical Specialist, Rehabilitation
   Irene Walker Johnson Institute of
      Rehabilitation
   Washington University School of
      Medicine
   St. Louis, MO

Definition

Your kidneys have a lot of work to do, 'cause normal kidney functions include eliminating your body's waste products; breaking down and eliminating medications and drugs; regulating body fluids, salts, and minerals; and regulating hormones that control healthy bones, blood count, and blood pressure. If your kidneys are unable to perform any of these jobs, you have a condition known as chronic renal disease.

The treatment of chronic renal disease includes a highly publicized technique in which your blood is "filtered" through a dialysis machine.

Specific Medical Considerations

If you have kidney disease, you may also have abnormal blood pressure (high or low), low blood count, or heart disease. You may be prone to weakness, nausea, and vomiting before or after dialysis. And you may have bone disease, muscle pain, muscle weakness, or pain or weakness because of abnormal nerve function. None of these factors, however, means that you should not exercise. In fact, regular exercise can be essential to your rehabilitation and treatment. It can, for example, help lower your blood pressure, as well as help normalize metabolism, body fluids, and blood count. But perhaps the most important benefit is that it makes you *feel* better. When you exercise, *you,* and not the "machine," are in charge!

Common Psychological or Behavioral Barriers to Exercise

Sue Caine, director of the National Kidney Foundation of Eastern Missouri & Metro East, summed it up pretty well: "The most significant psychological effect of end stage renal disease is the tendency of the patients and those around them (friends, family and government agencies) to consider them completely disabled. Dialysis patients are individuals with a persistent disorder that requires regular treatment. But when everybody adopts the attitude that they are 'chronically ill and disabled,' many otherwise healthy dialysis patients feel that they can't or shouldn't exercise. But the more they don't exercise, the more likely that they will become *truly* disabled."

Okay, you'd like to exercise, but you don't have time, right? You work all day, have a family to take care of, need a little recreation, and still have to squeeze in a trip to the hospital three times a week. Don't give me that old excuse! Regular exercise can help delay the onset of some of the metabolic and cardiovascular complications of your disease, and that alone ought to make it a major priority. But if you need another reason, exercise *with* your family AND have a lot of fun and recreation at the same time.

Specific Nutritional Concerns

You're gonna need to pay particular attention to the amount of fluid that you drink, and to the amount of sodium, potassium, calcium, phosphorus, and protein in your diet. This can be a very individual matter, so if you're not seeing a dietitian now, ask your physician to recommend one who's specially trained in renal disease.

Specific Precautions for a Program of General Exercise

You need to consult with your doctor before beginning your exercise program. Specifically, he or she will need to check your cardiovascular status and be certain that your blood pressure is well controlled. Any exercise will need to be carefully planned if you have poorly controlled hypertension, congestive heart failure, angina pectoris, irregular heart rhythm, an abnormal stress test, an electrolyte imbalance, heart-valve disease, severe bone disease or any other musculoskeletal disorder, symptomatic peripheral vascular disease or cerebral arteriosclerosis, severe or painful neuropathy, or severe anemia. That sounds like a lot, but most of you won't have those conditions. Only your doctor can tell, so go for that checkup!

Once you get the medical okay to begin, think about past exercise patterns. If this is the first time in twenty years, start with a few exercises, pay close attention to any changes in your body, and progress slowly as you feel stronger. A few minutes of exercise each day is much better than an hour-long session once a week!

Concentrate on exercises that maintain and increase flexibility and general muscle tone. (This would include the warm-up and the stretching and relaxation exercises in Chapter Three.) Any aerobic program should be developed gradually and with supervision.

Warning Signs of Physical Overextension

Dr. Wendy Weinstock Brown gave me some very specific signs for you to look for. Immediately STOP exercising if you:

"become severely short of breath,
become nauseated or dizzy,
develop chest pain or discomfort,
develop severe muscle pain,
become severely fatigued,
develop a rapid heartrate (faster than your doctor has determined is safe for you), or
develop an irregular heart rhythm."

Additionally, Dr. Brown told me, "Exercise which compromises vascular access must be avoided. For example, ankle circles must not be done if the patient has an access site at the ankle. And exercise in the first few hours after hemodialysis might be associated with bleeding, extreme fatigue or fainting."

If you follow the doctor's precautions, the benefits of exercise are many. As Dr. Brown concluded, "Regular exercise may delay or even avert the onset of many complications of chronic renal failure and thus, improve longevity. And it most certainly can improve your quality of life!"

SCHIZOPHRENIA AND MANIC DEPRESSION

THE MENTAL HEALTH ASSOCIATION
MHA IN LOS ANGELES COUNTY
930 GEORGIA ST., LOS ANGELES, CA 90015

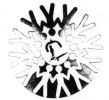

Consultant:

John Siegel
—Director
   Community Support Services
   The Mental Health Association in Los
      Angeles County
   Los Angeles, CA

Definition

You may wonder why mental illness is included in a book about physical disabilities. But the actual symptoms of disorders such as schizophrenia and manic depression prevent patients from keeping their bodies in top physical condition.

Patients with the chronic form of schizophrenia, for example, are usually isolated and withdrawn. Self-motivation for any activity, including exercise, is very low, and in severe cases, schizophrenic patients can experience hallucinations, delusions, and paranoia.

The major symptom of manic depression is extreme mood swings. A patient will cycle between feeling depressed (or even suicidal) and being overexcited and grandiose. Periods of enormous energy and ability are followed by periods of total inactivity. A patient may begin a program of exercise one day and be totally incapable of following it the next.

Specific Medical Considerations

When mental illness is managed with medication, that treatment can in itself prevent activities like exercise. This is because major tranquilizers often produce side effects like muscle rigidity, drowsiness, and even spasms.

Common Psychological or Behavioral Barriers to Exercise

John Siegel, director of Community Support Services for The Mental Health Association in Los Angeles County, tells me that the very pattern and discipline of a regular exercise program may be the main reason you choose not to exercise. He suggests approaching exercise gradually and with flexibility. Try an exercise with lots of variety, and for heaven's sake, don't count everything. Taking a walk, slow stretching to music, or dancing are also very good ways to begin. As you see your body responding, you're going to be encouraged to keep it up.

Warning Signs of Physical Overextension

As you may have observed in your own behavior, *mental* overextension is more likely than physical stress. When this happens, you probably just stop exercising. Sometimes, when it seems really stressful, you may even experience unrealistic fear of physical injury or pain. If you find yourself making lots of really terrific, fantastic excuses for *not* exercising, then you may be in this situation.

I asked John how he would encourage or motivate someone with mental illness to follow a program of exercise: "The same as anyone else. The important idea is to exercise daily at a convenient time and to slowly build interest and stamina. Most importantly, doing exercise with someone else can really help."

SHORT STATURE

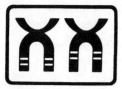

THE GENETICS INSTITUTE

Consultant:

E. Robert Wassman, Jr., M.D.
—Associate Director,
  The Genetics Institute
  Alhambra, CA
—Trustee
  Billy Barty Foundation

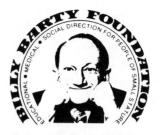

Consultant:

Martha Undercoffer
—Executive Director
  Billy Barty Foundation
  North Hollywood, CA

Definition

The term "short stature" is a relative one, and the degree of disability (if any) is also relative. Medical experts generally consider any adult under four feet ten inches to be of short stature. This group is further divided into people with *proportionate* short stature (this can be due to a hormonal imbalance, or it can simply mean that everybody else in your family is short) and *disproportionate* short stature (generally including what the lay public calls dwarfism). Most people of short stature have very little trouble doing anything they want to do. I know, 'cause a lot of high-achieving people that I look up to are shorter than four feet ten inches. And if you are of short stature, exercise is just as important for your heart and body as it is for anyone else's. But there are some special medical challenges for people with dwarfism, and these challenges need to be considered when you plan your program of exercise.

Specific Medical Considerations

If you have one of the many different types of dwarfism, there are two major medical considerations for you. The first is joint mobility. People with some forms of dwarfism may have a limited range of motion in some joints. (Usually, these are the shoulder and hip joints.) This means that your exercises must be carefully planned so you won't overextend an affected joint. Second, people with other types of dwarfism need to be very cautious about possible injury to the spinal column. Some people, for example, have a tendency to arthritis, and so jogging can be especially harmful. Others may need to avoid excessive neck movement. The exercises most often cited as being dangerous are jumping, wrestling, tumbling, diving, and overhead weight lifting, but you should check with your physician before beginning any specific exercise program.

Common Psychological or Behavioral Barriers to Exercise

This one's really simple, folks. The most common barrier is in the minds of people who think that ability has something to do with size. Dr. E. Robert Wassman (a very smart man who works at The Genetics Institute, is a trustee for the Billy Barty Foundation, and teaches pediatrics at the Harbor/UCLA Medical Center) put it this way: "The majority of individuals with short stature are extremely capable of coping with the physical limitations of the world around them. However, frustration and depression are not unknown when coping with the unwillingness of the 'average sized' world to accept their capabilities as complete human beings. The impact of this can lead to insecurities about appearing in public places such as exercise rooms or health clubs, where a great deal of attention is focused on the 'perfect body.'"

Amen, Dr. Wassman!

Now, this is where I come in—'cause I've spent the last twelve years of my life teaching people how to eat and exercise and I can tell you with no reservations, there *are no* perfect bodies. Absolutely none! There are perfect hearts and souls, but perfect bodies?? No way.

Specific Nutritional Concerns

The prime nutritional concern for *all* people of short stature is weight control. Trust me, I know a lot about this one, too. You look at one of those tall thin people who eats an entire pecan pie during coffee break and life definitely does not seem fair. So what else is new? Maybe when we all get to heaven, food will have no calories. But for now, we eat less and we move more.

Specific Precautions for a Program of General Exercise

Obviously, any specific precautions must be discussed with your doctor after he or she has analyzed your past medical history. But also use your good common sense. If you have recently experienced fractures, surgery (hip or spinal surgery is common for adults with dwarfism), or if one or more of your joints has either a limited or excessive range of motion, you need to adjust your exercise plan. Generally, though, you need to follow precautions similar for anyone else:

—Avoid overhead lifting of weights or excessively vigorous jumping.

—Never exercise beyond a point of pain or extreme fatigue.

—Start slowly and gradually increase the time you exercise.

—Exercise on a regular basis instead of a once-a-month sprint to the finish line.

And by the way, Dr. Wassman tells me that because swimming and bicycling allow movement with a relatively low gravitational pull on affected bones and joints they are *outstanding* daily exercises for anyone of short stature.

Warning Signs of Physical Overextension

Stop exercising if you experience a popping or slippage of a hypermobile (loose) joint, back pain, pain radiating into your legs, numbness, a "sleeping" sensation in your feet or hands, or any sense that you cannot catch your breath.

SICKLE-CELL DISEASE

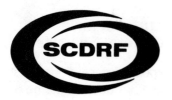

Consultants:

Ellen V. Jones, B.S.
—Education Director

Spencer C. Woods, D.P.A.
—Executive Director

L. Julian Haywood, M.D.
—Chairman
    Scientific & Research Committee

Patricia Corley, R.N.
—Summer Camp Nurse
    Comprehensive Sickle Cell Center

Cage S. Johnson, M.D.
—Summer Camp Medical Director
    Sickle Cell Disease Research
        Foundation
    Los Angeles, CA

Definition

Ellen Jones, education director for the Sickle Cell Disease Research Foundation, told me that this is a very misunderstood disease. Its cause is genetic and it comes from the presence of gene mutations that produce abnormal red blood cells. In the United States, most cases of sickle-cell disease occur among Afro-Americans. Approximately one in twelve blacks carries a single sickle-cell gene (a condition called sickle-cell trait), while approximately one in 500 black children has the *two* sickle-cell genes necessary to cause the disease. Scientists now believe that the abnormal sickle-cell gene arose among black populations in Africa as a protective mechanism against malaria, but sickle-cell anemia also affects people of Greek, Arabian, Maltese, Sicilian, Sardinian, and Turkish descent.

There are several clinical variants of the disease, ranging from very mild to severe anemia. Individuals with sickle-cell trait do not have the disease, but they're carriers of the sickle gene. If two sickle gene carriers marry, each child has a one in four chance of inheriting the disease.

Sickle-cell disease gets its name from the abnormal shape of the red blood cell. After oxygen is released from the cell, it assumes a sickle shape. In this irregular shape, the cell only lives for eight to fifteen days. The irreversibly sickled cell is so fragile that it is easily destroyed while passing through your body's small blood vessels. The rapid destruction of red blood cells also means that your bone marrow must be produced at a drastically increased rate. Even so, your body is unable to produce enough red blood cells to maintain normal levels, and so you get anemia.

Most individuals with sickle-cell disease are diagnosed shortly after birth. However, there are some who are diagnosed later in life (usually after severe complications).

Specific Medical Considerations

The irregular shape causes sickle cells to "clog up" at vessel intersections much like a log jam. The end result is extreme pain, often so bad that you must be hospitalized. And when blood vessels become clogged with sickle cells, circulation blockage causes what is known as a sickle-cell crisis. Besides the pain, other symptoms may result from reduced circulation and oxygen. These can include circulation disorders (especially in the abdomen, hands, feet, and bones); leg ulcers, various problems within your heart, kidney, and nervous system; increased risk of infection; fatigue; dehydration; jaundice; and delayed puberty.

Specific Precautions for a Program of General Exercise

The function of your red blood cells is to take oxygen from your lungs and distribute it to all parts of your body. Sickle-cell disease interferes with this basic function, and so extreme exercise requiring lots of oxygen may be inadvisable. But you still should do other kinds of exercise. Not only will appropriate exercise (done only after your doctor's okay) give you better overall physical conditioning, but it is also a perfect way to release anxiety, frustration, and stress. These three emotions are widely accepted as contributing factors to sickle-cell crisis. You might begin your exercise program with mild stretching exercises and gradually add activities such as jogging as your stamina builds.

Warning Signs of Physical Overextension

Assuming you have no other physical challenges, your warning signs are the same as for any other person. Follow a plan of warm-up, exercise, and cool-down. Stop exercising and rest if you experience any severe pain or discomfort, increasingly rapid or irregular heartrate, extreme fatigue, shortness of breath, dizziness, or nausea.

Dr. Cage S. Johnson told me that since all of the body's systems may be affected no two persons respond exactly alike. At this time, sickle-cell anemia is not curable, but with regular medical advice, problems related to the disease can be controlled and most of its complications can be managed successfully. Thus, many individuals with sickle-cell anemia lead active lives and maintain productive careers.

SPINA BIFIDA

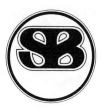

Consultant:

Kent Smith
—Executive Director
  Spina Bifida Association of America
  Chicago, IL

Consultant:

Richard E. Lindseth, M.D.
—Professor and Acting Chairman
  Department of Orthopedic Surgery
  Indiana University School of Medicine
  James Whitcomb Riley Hospital for
    Children
  Indianapolis, IN

OrthopædicHospital

Consultant:
Andrew Sew-Hoy, M.D.
Orthopaedic Hospital
Los Angeles, CA

Definition

Nobody yet knows the cause of spina bifida. What we do know is that it occurs when the spine does not properly close during fetal development. The results of this condition can include paralysis, loss of sensation in the lower limbs, and complications in the bowels and bladder. In addition, three-quarters of those children with spina bifida are also affected by a condition called hydrocephalus. (This is a blockage and accumulation of the fluids surrounding the brain and spinal cord, which if left uncontrolled can cause brian damage and mental retardation.)

The accumulated effects of spina bifida can result in severe developmental delays in social, emotional, vocational, and daily living skills.

For the past several years, I have been the national spokesperson for the Spina Bifida Association of America, and during that time I've witnessed the tremendous accomplishments of parents and families of children with this disorder. Increased medical and mechanical advancements in the treatment of spina bifida have been very dramatic. If you or your child has spina bifida and you are not a part of the up and active "mainstream," now is the time for you to "get with it!"

Common Psychological or Behavioral Barriers to Exercise

Sometimes the greatest psychological barrier a child with spina bifida encounters is the fears and concerns of his family members. Your child can and *should* follow an appropriate program of daily exercise. Only after *you* accept this idea can you communicate confidence and assurance to your child.

Specific Nutritional Concerns

Kids with spina bifida gain weight very easily. They have greatly reduced mobility, and some doctors even suspect a greatly reduced metabolic rate. More often, the real cause is the family that loves them the most. Please, don't use sugar and starchy snacks to say "I love you." Instead, show your love by teaching your child to prepare and enjoy healthful snacks, to recognize foods from the primary food groups, and to expect rewards of hugs and smiles instead of candy bars.

Disorders with vitamin C metabolism and constipation are also very common nutritional problems faced by spina bifida patients. You can help control these by including high levels of vitamin C (sometimes the doctor will even prescribe supplements) and a high-fiber diet (lots of vegetables and whole grain products).

Specific Precautions for a Program of General Exercise

Kent Smith, executive director of the Spina Bifida Association, suggests that you be particularly attentive to some key elements when planning exercises for your child. First, you should avoid those exercises (like back bends) that require severe trunk rotation. And it's extremely important that your child avoid any exercises that can put stress or pressure on his hip sockets. One way to do this is to try the exercise yourself and determine if the hip sockets are involved. And, of course, check with your physician if you are in doubt.

Children with shunts (a kind of release valve) for hydrocephalus should not participate in any exercise that involves twisting or spinning.

And finally, be alert to exercises involving the stomach muscles. These particular exercises are especially good for your child's weight control and overall fitness, but they can cause the bowels or bladder to empty involuntarily.

Warning Signs of Physical Overextension

If your child becomes nauseated, dizzy, or begins to lose his or her balance, you should stop exercising. Begin again the next day at a slower pace.

SPINAL CORD INJURY
(Quadriplegia and Paraplegia)

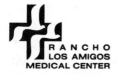

R A N C H O
LOS AMIGOS
MEDICAL CENTER

Consultants:

Marion B. Schoneberger, M.S., R.P.T.
—Physical Therapy Supervisor–
  Spinal Injury

Elizabeth Wyckoff–Benz, O.T.R.
—Occupational Therapy Supervisor,
    Pediatrics
  Rancho Los Amigos Medical Center
  Downey, CA

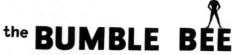

the **BUMBLE BEE**

An Exchange of Progress

Susanne McLean Owen
—Editor
  the Bumble Bee,
  An Exchange of Progress
  Pasadena, CA

Definition

The spinal cord carries information back and forth between your brain and the rest of your body. When it is injured, these messages are completely or partially interrupted and this in turn means a complete or partial loss of control and/or movement. Usually, the loss of function in all four limbs (arms and legs) is called quadriplegia and a loss of function in both legs is called paraplegia. In the most extreme cases, paralysis may involve the entire body so that a person cannot perform tasks without assistance.

Specific Medical Considerations

Everybody's an individual, and so the specifics of your spinal cord injury will have different results. For example, your injury may have caused instability in your spinal column, but much like a broken bone, it will heal in several months. During the healing process your movement will be restricted, but you'll gradually regain full use of your limbs. For other people, the damage may be permanent.

If you have an injury high on your spinal cord, you may need an artificial respirator to help you breathe, and/or you may be unable to cough independently. In both cases, medical problems such as colds and respiratory infections can be very serious. Bowel and bladder control (and resulting urinary and digestive infections) present another common medical challenge for a person with either paraplegia or quadriplegia. And finally, you have to work hard to prevent the skin breakdown and pressure ulcers that often occur because of long-term immobility.

Common Psychological or Behavioral Barriers to Exercise

Your biggest concern after a permanent injury may be how you feel about your dependence upon other people. It's all individual and can mean anything from minimal assistance with getting your wheelchair into your car to total dependence for all aspects of daily living. Marion Schoneberger, a physical therapist who works with people after spinal cord injury, told me, "The psychological impact of paralysis can be devastating, particularly during the first year or so following the injury. An individual may have no desire to pursue activities that are available. Many people with spinal injuries have the *ability* to exercise in some way—but no motivation or desire."

Motivation and desire are strengths you have to pull up from your own insides. Nobody can teach you or shame you or yell at you until you want to help yourself. But a lot of people with spinal injuries have found that regular exercise makes them feel better and function to their full potential.

Specific Precautions for a Program of General Exercise

Because certain conditions (like spinal fusions) require very specific precautions, talk to your doctor before beginning an exercise program. After you get the medical okay, start slowly and add repetitions only as your strength increases. Keep an eye out for areas on your body where the skin may be pinched or rubbed and you can't feel it.

Warning Signs of Physical Overextension

Often, a spinal cord injury will result in a condition called "autonomic dysreflexia." Simply put, this means that those neurological systems in your body that work "automatically" (things like your glands and even your heart) can suddenly stop working as well as they should. You should stop exercising and contact your doctor if you notice any of the symptoms of autonomic dysreflexia. These include excessive sweating, a flushing or blotching of your skin, goose bumps, chills without fever, a pounding headache, and an elevated blood pressure. (Note that the first two may be normal responses to vigorous exercise, but if accompanied by any of the other symptoms, call your doctor.)

And unless you have another physical challenge, you should just follow the warning signs appropriate for an able-bodied person: dizziness, shortness of breath, rapid or irregular heartbeat, excessive fatigue, or an actual decline in your muscle strength.

Last, but most important, get involved with other people again. I would recommend that you immediately get yourself a subscription to a terrific not-for-profit newsletter written and read by people with para- and quadriplegia. It's called *the Bumble Bee,* and it's edited by Susanne McLean Owen, 412 Woodward Blvd., Pasadena, CA 91107. In it you will read about other people who haven't given up on their bodies, reports of their progress, and tips on equipment and daily living skills.

When Sue Owen learned about this book, she had a message for you: "As the possibility of spinal nerve refunctioning becomes ever more probable, it's especially important that each of us do as much as we can to keep ourselves in good physical condition. If you happen to be one who has allowed his or her body to deteriorate, don't give up! START DOING SOMETHING ABOUT IT. The body has remarkable powers of renewal. But it can't do it without the cooperation of your head!"

STROKE

SHARP
MEMORIAL HOSPITAL

Consultants:

Helen Linn, R.N., B.S.N., C.R.R.N.
—Coordinator of CVA Services
   Sharp Rehabilitation Center

And the members of the
   Interdisciplinary Stroke Team
   Sharp Rehabilitation Center
Debbie Moore, R.T.R.
Barbara Johnson Ulrey, B.S., O.T.R.
Susan Edwards, B.S., O.T.R.
Ellen D. Morey, B.S., R.P.T.
Patricia R. Branigan, P.T. Assistant
Lisa Lowery, R.T. R.
Anita M. Pallai, B.S., O.T.R.
Mary Frances Gross, A.A., C.O.T.A.
Ann Martinez, R.P.T.
Sharp Memorial Hospital
San Diego, CA

Vernon Nickel, M.D.
—Medical Director

Bruce C. Baxley, Ph.D.
—Clinical Psychologist

Joanne G. Hein, M.S., C.C.C.
—Speech-Language Pathologist

Constance I. Lyford
—Associate Administrator

Joel M. Kunin, M.D.
—Director of Stroke Services

Janet Fisher-Gurr, R.N., B.S.N.
—CVA Lead Nurse

Esther Walsh, B.S, R. D.
—Clinical Dietitian

Definition

A stroke (also called a CVA for cerebrovascular accident) occurs when the blood supply to a specific part of the brain is interrupted by a blockage or hemorrhage (ruptured artery). Without this blood supply, nerve cells in the affected area can no longer communicate with the body parts they normally control. The site of a stroke determines which kinds of disabilities each person may experience, but some of the more common are paralysis on one half of the body or the impaired movement of either an arm or a leg; poor sitting or standing balance; problems with walking, coordination, touch, and sensation; and disorders with swallowing, speech, understanding, memory, judgment, perception, or vision.

Helen Linn, coordinator of Stroke Services for Sharp Memorial Hospital, also tells me that after a stroke the brain may "repair" some of its blood supply system or other areas of the brain may take over the work of the damaged cells. This makes the recovery of each person a very individual matter. However, with intense rehabilitation (including lots of exercise), many stroke-affected people regain function, learn to compensate, and soon develop much more independence. (Aren't you continually amazed at what brains can do? I am.)

Specific Medical Considerations

The effects of a stroke are always individual. And rehabilitation can be affected by so many other conditions (the aging process, previous health habits, lifestyle, and accompanying diseases such as diabetes and cardiovascular and respiratory disorders). So your first step before planning any exercise program is to see your physician. This way the two of you can rule out any specific movements that could interfere with your recovery.

Common Psychological or Behavioral Barriers to Exercise

Although a stroke has usually been silently building for a long time, when it comes it's sudden and dramatic. This kind of event can turn your world upside down. And the "emotional fallout" from that instant shock and trauma can get in the way of your recovery. Suddenly, you feel you're not what you were. Dr. Bruce Baxley, clinical psychologist at Sharp Memorial, talked about your post-stroke feelings like this: "Powerful emotional factors contribute to an overwhelming sense of *inability,* and this affects one's impetus to pursue a variety of activities—including exercise. Further, many people experience increased self-consciousness about their bodies following a CVA." He told me that many of you are embarrassed about the different ways your body works now, and that you may see exercise as some sort of competition—a competition that you'll lose. But none of those fears should control you now.

When you exercise—alone or in a group—forget about what perfect bodies are *supposed* to do. Nobody even knows what that is, anyway! Think instead about what exercise can do for you. The work and sweat you put into an exercise program today will come back to you a thousand times as you watch your body get stronger and more in control. Please, believe me—before long you'll forget all those fears and recognize only the gains you're making.

Specific Nutritional Concerns

It's true! Esther Walsh, registered dietitian with the CVA rehabilitation team, told me so: "Strokes commonly occur in people who have high blood pressure, diabetes and who are overweight. In addition, the American public is prone to oversalting food and to consuming large amounts of sugar, fats and meat. Changing these habits can significantly reduce the risk of a stroke." And even if you weren't overweight before the stroke, Esther says that it's very common for you to try to eat yourself out of the frustration you feel because of sudden immobility. Take it from a former frustrated fat person—it won't work! Now more than ever you need to study those points in Chapter Four, FOOD 4 LIFE, and learn about which foods keep you healthy and strong.

Specific Precautions for a Program of General Exercise

As you begin your exercise program, keep in mind these terrific suggestions from the specialists at the CVA Center of Sharp Memorial Hospital:

—Always start exercise with a warm-up period and finish by slowly cooling down.

—Plan your exercise according to your previous lifestyle. If, for example, you were a pretty sedentary person before the stroke, begin with five to ten minutes of exercise each day and slowly add exercises as you get stronger. The important thing is consistency, not setting endurance records.

—Wait at least one hour after eating before you exercise.

—Avoid any quick, jerky motions or any quick changes in body position. For example, don't rapidly rise from lying down to a sitting position.

—Be aware of any decrease in your normal sense of balance or field of vision.

—Don't exercise during times of extreme temperature, high humidity, or poor air quality.

—Avoid bending over and placing your head lower than your knees.

—If you have a weak shoulder or a shoulder joint separation, avoid shoulder motions of more than ninety degrees.

—Practice rhythmic breathing during exercise. This means breathing in during flexion of your muscle (usually at the beginning of a motion) and breathing out during relaxation (usually at the end of a motion). Never hold your breath during any activity.

—Finally and most important—have patience. Especially when you first begin your exercise program, the affected side of your body will not respond as quickly as will the side unaffected by your stroke. Enjoy each day and each accomplishment and soon the improvement will amaze you.

Warning Signs of Physical Overextension

Learn how to take your own pulse, and expect your heartrate to increase progressively during exercise. If your pulse should *decrease* with increased activity, STOP the exercise and immediately notify your physician.

Stop exercising if you experience any pain in your chest, neck, shoulder, or arm; shortness of breath; cramping or tightness in your calves; continuous pain in a joint; dizziness; cold sweaty forearms; sudden fatigue; or an irregular walk. As soon as you catch your breath, call your physician.

Janet Fisher-Gurr, CVA lead nurse at Sharp Memorial, had these final words for you: "The success of any exercise program (be it swimming, walking, calisthenics or bicycling) depends upon whether or not you enjoy and maintain it."

You know, she's absolutely right. Nobody's going to tell you that having a stroke is a good way to spend the afternoon. But don't forget, after that stroke you are first and foremost A SURVIVOR. So live and have fun with the activities you choose.

SYSTEMIC LUPUS ERYTHEMATOSUS

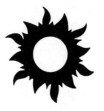

Consultants:

Roger Sturdevant
—Vice President

Ronald I. Carr, M.D., P.H.D.
—Member of the Medical Council
   The Lupus Foundation of America,
      Inc.
   St. Louis, MO

Definition

Lupus erythematosus (commonly called lupus) is a chronic connective tissue disease in which the body's organs are attacked and injured by the effects of a disordered immune system. Almost 1,000,000 Americans have this autoimmune process, thus making lupus more common than better-known diseases such as leukemia, muscular dystrophy, cerebral palsy, multiple sclerosis, or cystic fibrosis. The Lupus Foundation of America estimates that a new lupus patient is diagnosed every 10½ minutes! Women experience lupus at an almost 9-to-1 ratio over men.

The systemic form (also called SLE) may involve multiple tissues and organs, especially the skin, joints, kidneys, heart, lungs, central nervous system, and liver. A milder form, discoid lupus, can cause localized skin problems (most notably a butterfly-type rash across the bridge of the nose and cheeks).

SLE affects each person in a different way and to a different degree, but, generally, symptoms may include a skin eruption (typically the butterfly rash), weakness and lack of energy, diminished appetite and weight loss, frequent infections, as well as a chronic or recurrent low-grade fever. Joint pain or swelling simulating arthritis sometimes occurs. When the membranes around the internal organs become inflamed in some people with SLE, symptoms of heart or lung disease and gastrointestinal disturbances or abdominal pain may appear. Inflammation in the blood vessels to the bones can cause degeneration of bone and result in considerable pain. Some people with SLE also have spasms of the small vessels in the fingertips or toes after slight exposure to cold or even emotional stimulation. Another common symptom of SLE is hair loss leading to thinning of the hair and bald patches.

A person with SLE may bruise easily because of a reduced ability of the blood to clot properly. Moreover, kidney and neurological dysfunctions can occur and may even mimic the symptoms of other diseases and conditions. But perhaps the most intriguing symptom of lupus is a striking sensitivity to the sun (or, in rarer cases, sensitivity to fluorescent lights). Almost 40 percent of the people with lupus find that sunlight aggravates the illness.

This is a systemic disease and that means that every system of the body can be affected—but it's important to realize that with proper treatment the severity of the symptoms and complications of lupus can usually be reduced or even prevented.

The Lupus Foundation of America believes that some doctors go overboard in stressing only the disastrous aspects of lupus. When treating the disease, some doctors even prescribe rest and minimal exertion. In reality, the patient should be encouraged to be as active as possible (including normal employment).

A program of conditioning exercises that promote muscle tone (like walking, swimming, and bicycling) should increase the overall feeling of well-being. And there is no reason why individuals gifted with athletic ability in one or more sports should not continue to enjoy them, as long as they protect themselves from the sun and from exhaustion.

Not only may inactivity be unnecessary, but it can also lead to increased weakness, boredom, and time for self-pity. All of these are detrimental to both the person with SLE and his or her family.

Specific Precautions for a Program of General Exercise

Because of the variety of effects of SLE, you should plan your daily exercise program only after checking with your physician. Generally, you should start slowly and add exercises as your stamina increases. When exercising, follow a plan of warm-up, exercise, rest periods, exercise, and cool-down.

The idea that SLE is a fatal disease is one of the gravest misconceptions about this illness. The survival rate has increased dramatically, and the vast majority of children and young adults with SLE will not die from the disease. With improved methods of therapy on the horizon, an even better outlook will occur.

So it seems to me that it's time for you to stop living in the past and start working today for your new, thinner, and healthier future!

TOURETTE SYNDROME

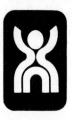

Consultant:

Ruth Dowling Bruun, M.D.
—Chairman
   Medical Committee
   Tourette Syndrome Association
—Director
   Movement Disorder Clinic
   Payne-Whitney Clinic
   New York Hospital Medical Center
   New York, NY

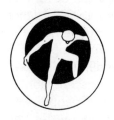

Consultant:

Abbey S. Meyers
—Director
   Government and Industry Liaison
      Committee
   National Organization for Rare
      Disorders
   New York, NY

Definition

Tourette syndrome is a nondegenerative neurological movement disorder that usually begins between the ages of two and sixteen. No one knows the exact cause of TS, but it appears to be triggered by a chemical imbalance in the brain. People with this syndrome exhibit varying degrees of involuntary movements, such as tics and twitches (*i.e.,* rapid eye blinking, shoulder shrugging, head jerking, facial twitches, etc.). In addition, some people with TS make repetitive involuntary sounds, such as throat clearing, grunting, sniffing, or shouting.

Specific Medical Considerations

If you have TS, you may be taking medications such as haloperidol or pimozide. These drugs sometimes inhibit the natu-

ral "cooling down" process of your body, so when you exercise, be especially careful that you don't become overheated.

Sometimes the medication given for TS can make you feel tired and listless. If this is true for you, the schedule and pattern of *regular* exercise can be just the thing to help you "get up and go."

Common Psychological or Behavioral Barriers to Exercise

Most people with TS have a great deal of excess energy. In children this is often defined as "hyperactivity," and in adults it is described with phrases like "inner tension." It probably seems to you that you *must* be in constant motion. When discussing this common behavioral pattern, Dr. Ruth Dowling Bruun, chairman of the Medical Committee for the Tourette Syndrome Association, said, "Exercise usually helps relieve tension and promote relaxation. And so most people with TS are enthusiastic participants in athletic endeavors. Some, however, find that the excitement of competitive sports increases TS symptoms and so prefer instead to engage in more solitary forms of exercise."

So if you're somebody who likes solitary (or small-group, noncompetitive) exercise and if this TS appendix entry is the only one you need to read, guess what? Any exercise in our book can be a part of your personal exercise program. So enjoy!

Specific Nutritional Concerns

Some people with TS are very sensitive to central nervous system stimulants such as caffeine, so avoid excessive amounts of cola drinks, chocolate, and coffee. (And I'm sure that your physician has already warned you about taking over-the-counter antihistamines since most of them also contain stimulants.)

Warning Signs of Physical Overextension

If you're taking *any* medication, it's important for you to watch for dizziness, faintness, shortness of breath, or palpitations (that's when your heart feels like it's going to beat its way right through your chest). If these sensations occur, stop exercising, go to a cool place, and relax. This doesn't mean that you should stop exercising forever and for all time. Forget it. You're not going to get off that easily! All you need to do is to talk to your physician about modifying the specific exercises you've included in your plan.

I asked Dr. Bruun if she had any other comments for you and she said, "Exercise can be a constructive way to use the excessive energy you may find so burdensome. However, practice caution when taking medication and have any exercise program approved by your physician."

VISUAL IMPAIRMENT

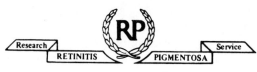

"Fighting Blindness"

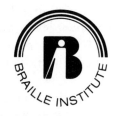

Consultant:

Helen Harris
—President
  Retinitis Pigmentosa International
  Woodland Hills, CA

Consultants:

Sara Ingber

Donald I. Macnab-Stark
—Youth Director
  Braille Institute
    Youth Center
  Los Angeles, CA

PREVENT BLINDNESS.

Consultant:

Freda M. Hinsche
—Executive Director
  National Society to Prevent Blindness
    Southern California
  Orange, CA

Definition

Visual impairment is a very broad term. In fact, most of us have less than perfect eyesight at some point in our lives. But now I'm talking about exercise for those people with visual impairment from conditions such as glaucoma, cataracts, having one eye, keratitis, toxic optic neuritis, retinal hemorrhages, diabetes, retinal tears, and temporary effects of postoperative healing. Legal blindness (as a result of any of these conditions) is defined as less than 20/200 corrected vision in the better of your two eyes. That means that you are able to see at twenty feet what other people can see at 200.

Specific Medical Considerations

When your vision is impaired (even temporarily), the *rest* of your body *still* needs exercise. But specific visual challenges can mean specific precautions for specific movements, and so you must check with your doctor before beginning exercise. For example, a visual impairment resulting from bleeding within the eye (such as from diabetes) may mean that you shouldn't bend over from the waist or do exercises like push-ups. If you have a detached retina or a retinal hemorrhage, you probably shouldn't exercise using quick, sharp movements of your head. Studies show that people with glaucoma have an unusually high buildup of fluid within the eye and, therefore, should not use gravity boots or hang upside down for periods of time. Finally, because they have diminished depth perception, people with vision in only one eye need to be very careful when choosing an exercise with rapid movements.

Common Psychological or Behavioral Barriers to Exercise

Once you've decided to exercise, the biggest challenge is usually simple logistics. Helen Harris, president of Retinitis Pigmentosa International, put it this way: "People with impaired vision love to exercise, but it is often the first thing that is lost as sight begins to fail. Initially there is the fear that quick movement will result in injury, and so blind and partially sighted persons stop moving quickly and thus lose body tone. Moreover, while special classes and exercise programs would greatly help, the visually impaired cannot take advantage of these opportunities if they cannot even get there. Transportation can become a major problem. A sighted guide must take the time to escort a blind or partially sighted person to such a program."

Helen then reminded me that once you get to an exercise class or one of those terrific outdoor fitness courses, sighted participants and instructors often forget the simple things like verbally announcing exercise instructions and showing you where the bathrooms are.

All of this dependence upon sighted escorts can really be a pain—not to mention what it does to your confidence and self-esteem!

Let's face it, things don't always follow storybook plots. If you have the opportunity to attend a well-organized group exercise program, that's wonderful. Enjoy yourself and get busy building that strong, firm body. But if that's not going to happen, your body can still turn to mush while you sit around waiting for a ride to the gym. Take charge of your exercise program yourself. First, you need a plan. Start with that talk with your doctor. Ask about any movements you should avoid and for exercises that may fit your individual needs. Pick a regular time each day for your exercise program, push the furniture against the wall to clear a large space, have a slow run-through to be sure you're not going to kick the sofa or something, turn on some music, and get on with it! Before long, you're gonna feel better and you're gonna BE better.

If you are the parent of a child with blindness or severe visual impairment, you have to be particularly careful about being overprotective. You want your child to be safe, but you also want him or her to be secure, happy, and free. Planning and participating in a regular exercise program can help. Make this an opportunity for your child to explore and learn not only about his environment but about his abilities as well.

Warning Signs of Physical Overextension

Just like everybody else, you need to start out slowly and add exercises as your body gets back in the swing of things. If you have any other medical condition (such as diabetes), be alert to excessive sweating, dizziness, heart palpitations, cold moist skin, or extreme fatigue. If any of these sensations should occur, stop exercising and contact your doctor for a review of your exercise plan.

Don Macnab-Stark works with young blind people at the Braille Institute Youth Center in Los Angeles. He summed it up like this: "If you look after your body, your whole life will benefit. You'll feel better about yourself, and this will be reflected in everything you do."

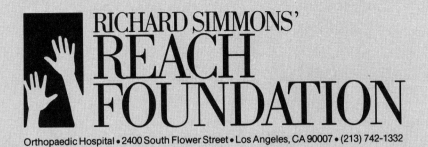

RICHARD SIMMONS'
REACH
FOUNDATION

Orthopaedic Hospital • 2400 South Flower Street • Los Angeles, CA 90007 • (213) 742-1332

If you would like to learn more about the Reach Foundation, or if you would like to help us with our work, please write:

Lawrence R. Apodaca, Executive Director
Richard Simmons' Reach Foundation
Orthopaedic Hospital
P.O. Box 60132, Terminal Annex
Los Angeles, CA 90060